CANDIDA
CLEANSE

CANDIDA CLEANSE

*The 21–Day Diet
to Beat Yeast and Feel Your Best*

SONDRA FORSYTH

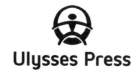

Ulysses Press

Published in the U.S. by:
Ulysses Press
P.O. Box 3440
Berkeley, CA 94703
www.ulyssespress.com

ISBN13: 978-1-61243-305-9
Library of Congress Control Number: 2013957238

Printed in Canada by Marquis Book Printing

10 9 8 7 6 5 4 3 2 1

Acquisitions Editor: Katherine Furman
Project Editor: Keith Riegert
Managing Editor: Claire Chun
Editor: Susan Lang
Proofreader: Elyce-Berrigan-Dunlop
Index: Sayre Van Young
Production: Lindsay Tamura
Cover design: Double R Design
Cover artwork: © Jenny Solomon/shutterstock.com

Distributed by Publishers Group West

NOTE TO READERS: This book has been written and published strictly for informational and educational purposes only. It is not intended to serve as medical advice or to be any form of medical treatment. You should always consult with your physician before altering or changing any aspect of your medical treatment. Do not stop or change any prescription medications without the guidance and advice of your physician. Any use of the information in this book is made on the reader's good judgment and is the reader's sole responsibility. This book is not intended to diagnose or treat any medical condition and is not a substitute for a physician.

Contents

Phase 3: Maintenance
(Keeping Candida in Check for a Lifetime)

Introduction

The Fungus That's Now Among Us—and Why

Remember the schoolyard taunt "There's a fungus among us?" The chant was typically followed by a chorus of "Kill it before it multiplies!" Those bullies on the playground might as well have been talking about the fungus *Candida albicans*. It starts out as a friendly yeast among the beneficial microbes in your intestines but morphs into a meanie if you indulge in what is called the Western diet—a diet high in sugar, red meat, white flour, and processed foods. The transformation from benevolent yeast to nasty fungus might also happen if you take certain medications such as antibiotics and oral contraceptives or you undergo chemotherapy. Whatever the cause, the result is a condition called Candida overgrowth, which can bring on myriad health problems.

1

First, the Good News!

The main strategy you have to follow is to starve it by cutting out the foods it needs to survive. That's the good news. The even better news is that because those foods just happen to be the same ones that are bad for your health in general, the Candida Cleanse diet will boost your vitality and give you a wonderful feeling of overall well-being.

One thing leads to another: When you cut out sugar and white flour, that means most processed foods are out—but you still need to eat, so you go for fresh foods instead of processed foods and whole grains instead of white flour, and you quit craving sugar. The result? You feel terrific—and virtually rejuvenated! Imagine waking up in the morning refreshed and invigorated, ready to take on the joys and challenges of the day ahead instead of dragging yourself out of bed with aches and pains and a general sense of malaise. Convinced? Great!

But what next? What exactly should your diet consist of? If you search for "Candida" on the Internet, you'll get tens of millions of results. Change the search to *"Candida albicans"* and you'll reduce the results to a few million. "Candida cleanse" will net you about a couple of million choices, and "Candida cleanse diet" will yield nearly that many possibilities. I'm pretty sure that you don't want to wade through all those results. Fortunately, this book organizes all the important facts available about Candida overgrowth and presents them to you in an easy-to-digest form. You'll find concise yet comprehensive information about diet and lifestyle changes that can get your system back to normal after the good little yeast in your gut morphs into an opportunistic pathogen.

You don't have to resort to liquid diets or colonics to beat back the Candida fungus. Instead, the Candida Cleanse is a very easy-to-follow three-phase program: Phase 1 is the powerful 21-day cleanse, which kills the fungus while allowing you plenty of healthy food to eat; Phase 2 continues to starve the fungus as you add back more foods to your eating regimen; and Phase 3 is your diet for life. Honestly, it's simple—and you won't feel deprived!

Okay, so you know you *can* defeat Candida overgrowth. Thus far I've given you the bare essentials of how and why the overgrowth happens, so now let's get into detail. Why *does* Candida go on the rampage?

Gut Microbes out of Balance

Candida isn't inherently a bad guy. In its one-celled state, it's a valuable yeast that helps absorb nutrients and protects your intestinal tract from infections. Candida turns into a villain only when your "gut flora" (the microbes in your intestines) are thrown off balance. Overgrowth is simply the phenomenon of the benign one-celled yeast transforming into its menacing form—with long filaments penetrating mucous surfaces and becoming invasive. This overgrowth happens because the bacteria that keep Candida in check have been depleted.

One result of the overgrowth can be the miserably itchy genital infections that plague both men and women. Another common problem is oral overgrowth, known as thrush. Beyond that, a wide range of disorders, including chronic pain, irritable bowel syndrome, anxiety, and depression may result when Candida runs amok.

WARNING!

Invasive candidiasis and candidemia, a form of invasive candidiasis, are potentially fatal bloodstream infections. According to the Centers for Disease Control, the infections are extremely rare in people without risk factors such as a compromised immune system, but they are the fourth most common hospital-acquired bloodstream infections in the United States. Symptoms include fever and chills. The diagnosis is made with a blood culture. Immediate medical attention and treatment with antibiotics are essential.

Antibiotics Overprescribed

One reason for the high incidence of Candida overgrowth is that doctors vastly overprescribe antibiotics for ailments that don't call for these medications. A study led by the University of California, San Francisco found that in the United States between 2007 and 2009 broad-spectrum drugs aimed at a wide range of bacteria—rather than narrow-spectrum drugs aimed at a limited range—accounted for the majority of antibiotic use among people who were not hospitalized. Not only that, but more than a quarter of the prescriptions were for conditions against which antibiotics aren't even effective.

The result is that the gut flora of the hapless patient who swallows this unnecessary medication is thrown out of kilter—giving Candida just the opportunity it needs to dominate and transform from good yeast to menacing fungus.

Taking antibiotics, whether you really needed them or for no good reason, may be at least one of the reasons for your Candida overgrowth. But take heart! The Candida Cleanse can correct the problem by depriving the fungus of the nutrients it needs to survive.

Here's a real-life story about Sharon, a victim of what has been dubbed "French bread thumb":

While cutting a loaf of bread I sliced into my left thumb. Instinctively, I stuck my thumb in my mouth and sucked on the wound. Bad move! As I later learned, the human mouth is rife with germs that can cause harm—unlike animal saliva, which can actually promote healing. Because I was in a rush to complete the preparations for my dinner party, I simply ran cold water over my thumb and didn't bandage the cut.

The party went well, and later I fell into a peaceful sleep only to wake up at 3 a.m. with throbbing pain in my thumb. I tiptoed into the bathroom to avoid waking my husband and flicked on the light. To my horror, I saw that my thumb was grossly swollen. Worse yet, a red line was moving up my arm. I woke my husband, who called 911, and in short order I found myself in the hospital hooked to intravenous antibiotics to forestall the ominous possibility that I could die of sepsis, or blood poisoning.

Obviously, I lived through the ordeal and a couple of days later went home with a prescription for oral antibiotics. By the time I finished my course of antibiotics, I had all the symptoms of a full-blown case of Candida overgrowth.

At least Sharon actually needed the antibiotics to save her life. Tom, who recounts his story here, had a very different experience. There was no reason for him to take the antibiotics he received.

> I developed a nagging little cough one winter,
> which in retrospect I believe was from an allergy
> to dust I breathed in while cleaning out the attic.
> However, my doctor said that I probably had
> chronic bronchitis and prescribed antibiotics. My
> cough didn't get better, but I did start feeling the
> general malaise that I later learned is so common
> with Candida overgrowth.

The encouraging news is that both Sharon and Tom were able to beat back Candida overgrowth by following the cleanse. Sharon had this reaction:

> I honestly feel better now than I did before my
> little kitchen accident. I never thought of myself
> as someone who didn't eat healthy, but I was
> actually consuming a lot of processed food and
> sugar without even realizing it. I'm obviously glad
> I didn't die from the blood poisoning, but I'm also
> glad the whole incident happened because the
> Candida Cleanse changed my life for the better.

Tom had a similar reaction:

> I used to pretty much eat "guy food." You know,
> wings and beer for the Super Bowl, plenty of meat
> and potatoes, lots of fried stuff, and not much in
> the way of veggies and fruits. Now I'm eating right,
> my cough is gone, and I'm a new man!

The Unhealthy Western Diet

Of course, antibiotics and other pharmaceuticals such as oral contraceptives and chemotherapy drugs are far from the only causes of what is probably a Candida pandemic. A major perpetrator is the Western diet, which is high in sugar, red meat, saturated fats, white flour, and processed foods, and low in fresh fruits and vegetables, healthy fats, whole grains, seafood, and poultry. The antithesis is the Mediterranean diet, which happens to be high in those foods that are scarce in the Western diet.

Various studies—including one at the University of Athens, Greece, that followed more than 22,000 participants for more than 11 years—have shown that the Mediterranean diet promotes good health. That diet is very similar to the Candida Cleanse diet, which also calls for eating fresh fruits and vegetables, whole grains, onions, garlic, and olive oil, and—this is critical—cutting out sugar and processed foods.

These and numerous other studies confirm that we are indeed what we eat. So, no matter what has made you prone to Candida overgrowth, the Candida Cleanse will not only arm you to win the battle against the "fungus among us" but will also give you the best possible chance of living long and well.

Now, let's get down to the basics of Candida overgrowth. We're going to Candida school...

PART ONE

CANDIDA OVERGROWTH 101

Everything you need to know about the good-yeast-turned-menacing-fungus—plus what you should and shouldn't do to beat it back

1

Symptoms of Candida Overgrowth

Genital yeast infections and oral thrush are irrefutable symptoms. The list of other symptoms, however, is long and controversial in the opinion of many Western health care providers. Some indicators that could tip you off to Candida overgrowth include frequent throat clearing of excess mucus, a generalized itchy feeling, bad breath, adult-onset allergies, scaly skin, and an oddly pungent body odor. Many sufferers also mention fatigue and feeling "spacey." The reported symptoms—other than genital yeast infections and oral thrush—often don't respond to conventional treatments, so many doctors think that people reporting them are hypochondriacs.

One 50-something woman put it like this:

> When I went for my annual physical, I told the
> doc I had all these random aches and pains and I

was tired literally all the time no matter how much sleep I got. He kind of smiled and said I'm just getting older. Come on! I'm not that old! I was sick in some vague way that I just couldn't get the doctor to believe or understand. He gave me a clean bill of health and told me to come back in a year. I was so discouraged.

Then about a week later, I got what turned out to be my first ever vaginal yeast infection. It was itchy and there was this disgusting discharge that looked like cottage cheese so I went straight back to the doctor and he diagnosed it. He gave me antifungal cream. But he never put two and two together, like about how my overall feeling of ill health might be somehow connected to my yeast infection. It took a girlfriend to do that for me. I told her about my problems and she was like, honey, you have Candida overgrowth! I was blown away.

If that sounds familiar, you may well have Candida overgrowth. But that's only one scenario out of many. Here's a list of possible symptoms and conditions:

Adult-Onset Allergies

You may become sensitive to various foods and to airborne triggers such as ragweed for the first time in your life. One woman in her late 40s had recently been grabbing fast food for lunch and dinner because of a hectic new job. Then she went to a Memorial Day picnic at a state park and ended up having to leave because of a sudden sneezing fit and impossibly itchy eyes. She had never had this reaction before, but the allergy persisted until she did the Candida Cleanse.

Common food allergies that may come on as a result of Candida overgrowth include adverse reactions to wheat, corn, milk and some milk products (especially cow's milk), eggs, and nightshade vegetables such as potatoes, tomatoes, eggplant, and peppers.

Fatigue

Chronic fatigue syndrome, often dismissed as psychosomatic in Western medicine, can be a real health problem if you have Candida overgrowth. The sense of exhaustion is most often continuous, but it can get worse after you eat.

Tummy Troubles

You may frequently suffer from diarrhea, constipation, bloating, gas, stomach cramps, heartburn, or bouts of nausea. Babies may have colic.

Sugar Cravings

If you suddenly have an uncharacteristic urge to eat sweets, that may be a sign that your overgrown Candida is pleading for a meal.

Mood Swings

Women are no strangers to the erratic moods of premenstrual syndrome and menopause, but Candida overgrowth can vastly exacerbate these ups and down. Men can also experience unexplained mood swings as a result of Candida overgrowth. A key indicator is irritability with no apparent cause. In children, this may manifest itself as hyperactivity, attention deficit disorder, aggression, or sleep problems.

Headaches

From garden-variety temple pounders to full-blown migraines, headaches of all levels can affect Candida sufferers.

Confusion

No matter your age, you may have trouble concentrating and feel foggy and confused much of the time. I call this "Candida brain." Memory problems not unlike "senior moments" can be part of this syndrome too. You may experience one or more of these symptoms:

Slurred speech: You haven't had a drop to drink, but your speech is slurred as though you had multiple sclerosis. You may also have other MS-like symptoms such as impaired muscle coordination and blurry vision.

Depression and anxiety after eating: Experiencing the blues or feeling panicky after a meal are common reactions to Candida overgrowth.

Paranoia: The disconcerting sense that "they" are out to get you is a common neurological response when Candida proliferates.

Indecision: You may know on a rational level what the right course of action or the best choice is, but you feel strangely unable to follow through—so you simply sit there waffling.

Female Problems

Vaginal infections are the obvious condition, but women with Candida overgrowth may also have irregular or painful menstrual periods, frequent urinary tract infections, and even infertility issues. Watch out for rectal itching and burning too.

Guy Problems

Men can have rectal itching as well as jock itch. More serious problems include erectile dysfunction and a swollen, inflamed prostate gland due to a condition called prostatitis.

Respiratory Tract Troubles

You may have frequents colds and be prone to the flu, or you may simply have constant mucous congestion and postnasal drip. Other signs are frequent clearing of the throat and a nagging little cough that isn't "productive," meaning that it doesn't clear out mucus. Other more worrisome issues include asthma, bronchitis, and tonsillitis (even in adults).

Chronic ear infections: Children are especially prone to this problem but adults can have it as well. The ears are considered part of the respiratory tract because the Eustachian tube connects the middle ear to the pharynx.

Skin and Mouth Woes

Rashes and blisters in the groin, between fingers and toes, and under the breasts are common. Also typical are athlete's foot, hives, dry brownish patches, psoriasis, ringworm, toenail fungus, and patches of rough skin. In babies, cradle cap and diaper rash are problems.

Thrush: Creamy white patches on your tongue or throat and cracks at the corners of your mouth indicate this condition. Infants and children are prone to it as well.

General Malaise

Of all the symptoms of Candida overgrowth, the real tip-off is a general sense of malaise. You simply don't feel well. You wake up with no sense of being refreshed by a good night's sleep, and you may in fact experience sleep problems. If you're over 40 or 50, you may attribute this state of affairs to normal aging. But it's not about age! And if you're a fairly young person, you may feel older than your years and not know why. Also, no matter how many candles were on your last birthday cake, you may be eating what you think is a healthy diet and living a fairly healthy lifestyle but you're still constantly feeling under par. Here's how one man in his 40s described his experience with Candida overgrowth:

> I'm an avid outdoorsman and I have been active all my life—mountain climbing, hiking, kayaking, canoeing. Then when I hit 40, my whole system just seemed to slow down. I figured it was middle age catching up to me, but I got so depressed. My buddies and I would get to the put-in for a big kayaking trip with the promise of some epic first descents on waterfalls, and I would find myself wanting to quit and go back home. I was exhausted and the day hadn't even started. I also felt slightly nauseated. I'd think about all the energy and enthusiasm I had when I was younger and I couldn't believe that I suddenly felt like a worn-out codger.

> Finally at the start of one trip, I said I was going back home because I didn't feel well. My wife was in shock when I showed up at the house because she knew how much I always looked forward to kayaking. She got on the Internet and found out about Candida overgrowth. Bless her heart, she

started buying and cooking all the right foods for me and within a couple of months I was my old self again. I'm back out on the rivers running class IV whitewater and I feel fantastic. Oh, and our sex life is great again. I hadn't been very good in bed while I was so down and maybe that was part of what motivated my wife to research my problem. Hey, whatever it takes! I'm glad she did.

That's the toll that Candida overgrowth stealthily takes on your well-being. Don't settle for a lower quality of life. Embark on the Candida Cleanse and vow to follow it faithfully.

But first, read on to find out whether diagnostic tests can determine if you really do have Candida overgrowth.

2

Tests for Candida Growth

Are there tests for Candida overgrowth? The answer is "yes" and "maybe."

Visual Test for Candida

Let's start with the "yes" part first. If you suspect you have the oral Candida infection called thrush, just stick your tongue out and look in the mirror. A white coating should be obvious. You can go to the doctor for verification if you want to be absolutely sure, but only in some cases will a doctor order a lab test to look for underlying conditions that could make you more susceptible to oral thrush.

A visual test is also all that's needed to diagnose jock itch, the popular name for the genital Candida infection that guys get. For yeast vaginitis, you'll need to have a gynecologist do an exam with a speculum inserted into your vagina. However, you can also buy an over-the-counter test from your drugstore and use it yourself to rule out other possibilities such as bacterial vaginosis and trichomonia-sis. The distinctive symptom of vaginal yeast infection is pretty obvious: an odorless discharge that is white with curds. You may also have burning when you urinate and experience pain during sex.

Spit Test for Candida

Now, let's consider the "maybe" part. You can try the spit test. Leave a glass of water beside your bed and spit into it as soon as you wake up in the morning. If, after a few minutes, the spit looks like a web, you probably have overgrowth. Stool tests and blood tests can also detect Candida overgrowth, but they are not always definitive, *except in the case of the potentially lethal blood infections candidiasis and candidemia* (see page 4).

Candida Questionnaire

A Candida questionnaire is one of your best bets for learning whether you probably have Candida overgrowth. Homeopathic practitioners rely on questionnaires to diagnose what they call "leaky gut syndrome," in which the protective membrane in your intestines is weakened, allowing the overgrowth to escape and wreak havoc in your entire system. Here's a questionnaire based on the one devised by the late William G. Crook, M.D., author of the 1983 book *The Yeast Connection*, and modified to reflect more recent research. Dr. Crook's work is considered contro-

versial by many in the Western medical establishment, but
homeopathic practitioners maintain that it's valid.

- ❏ Have you ever taken antibiotics more than
  10 days at a time and/or several times a year?
  Examples are tetracycline for acne, and broad-
  spectrum antibiotics for urinary tract infections
  (UTIs or cystitis), bronchitis, or other infections.

- ❏ Have you ever taken birth control pills (oral
  contraceptives), especially for 2 years or more?

- ❏ Have you ever been pregnant?

- ❏ Have you ever taken oral steroids or had steroid
  injections or inhaled steroid treatments or used
  steroid eyedrops, whether for pain relief or
  asthma treatment? These drugs are also called
  corticosteroids. Examples include cortisone,
  prednisone, and dexamethasone.

- ❏ Have you ever taken anabolic steroids for athletic
  performance enhancement? Examples include
  oxymetholone and methandrostenolone, among
  others.

- ❏ Are you allergic to perfumes and other scented
  products?

- ❏ Does damp, chilly weather make your symptoms
  worse?

- ❏ Have you ever had athlete's foot?

- ❏ Have you ever had jock itch?

- ❏ Have you ever had vaginal yeast infections?

Tests for Candida Growth

❏ Have you ever had nail fungus?

❏ Do you have an extreme sweet tooth?

❏ Do you have intense carbohydrate cravings such as for bread or crackers?

❏ Do you have a general sense of lethargy?

❏ Does your memory sometimes fail you?

❏ Do you ever feel confused?

❏ Do you suffer from depression?

❏ Do you have bouts of numbness or tingling in your extremities?

❏ Do you have unexplained aches and pains?

❏ Are you sometimes bloated or gassy?

❏ Are you often constipated?

❏ Do you often have bouts of diarrhea?

❏ Have you lost your libido?

❏ Do you have erectile dysfunction?

❏ Do you have unusually painful menstrual periods?

❏ Is your vision sometimes blurry, possibly with spots before your eyes?

❏ Are you often irritable or jittery or do you suffer from mood swings for no apparent reason?

❏ Do you have trouble concentrating?

❏ Do you have frequent headaches?

❑ Do you sometimes feel dizzy or unsteady on your feet?

❑ Do you have rashes or generalized itching?

❑ Do you have indigestion or acid reflux?

❑ Is there sometimes mucus in your stools?

❑ Do you often have hemorrhoids?

❑ Is your mouth often dry?

❑ Does your breath have an odd, unpleasant odor?

❑ Do you have an oddly pungent body odor?

❑ Do you often have nasal congestion or postnasal drip?

❑ Do you often have a persistent, unproductive cough?

❑ Do you feel a frequent need to clear your throat?

❑ Do you have incontinence (bladder leakage), either the stress or the urge type?

❑ Do you have frequent ear infections, or did you as a child?

❑ Do you have metabolic syndrome or type 2 diabetes?

If you have even a few of these symptoms, the Candida Cleanse is definitely worth a try. As I mentioned earlier, the diet is so good for you that you'll feel better no matter what your complaints are. Here's how one woman in her early 40s put it:

I just took it for granted that I was slowing down because I had hit midlife. I would wake up every morning not feeling rested and I didn't have the energy I used to have. I also had food allergies I never experienced before and frequent bouts of sinusitis. Of course, I knew I wasn't taking very good care of myself because I was so stressed and busy as a single working mother, but I told myself I didn't have time to sit down to a decent lunch or do any more for breakfast than grab a power bar. Dinner was often fast food, which I knew was bad for my kids, but most evenings I was too wiped out to cook. Then my sister got on my case at a family reunion. She recommended a Candida diet and she said she was going to text me some reminders several times a day to keep me on the straight and narrow. She even went food shopping with me the following weekend.

Well, the results have been spectacular. Now I have plenty of get-up-and-go and I even started running. My kids feel better too! They are actually learning to cook and sometimes they have a healthy dinner waiting for me when I get home. This has been a win-win for me in every way. I highly recommend the diet!

With that encouraging testimony in mind, read on to learn the truth about antifungal medications and supplements.

3

Do I Need Antifungal Medication and Supplements?

As you'll see when we get to the diet itself, you shouldn't start taking antifungal oral medications or supplements until after the 21-day Candida Cleanse. That's when you might start to experience Candida "die-off," although some people experience die-off a little sooner and others don't have die-off at all. Die-off is a process explained in detail in Chapter 22. Some of your symptoms may seem worse and you could even have new ones. But this is because the cleanse is working! The diet is killing the fungus, and the dead fungus is releasing toxins. Please don't let this brief annoyance discourage you and cause you to go back to your old way of eating. You'll feel better in just a few days.

Relief for Vaginal Infections, Jock Itch, and Thrush

If you have a genital yeast infection—vaginal for the ladies and jock itch for the gentlemen—you want to stop that itching right away, regardless of which phase of the cleanse you're in. Fortunately, there are over-the-counter topical applications available. For jock itch, a common OTC treatment is terbinafine HCL, marketed as Lamisil. For yeast vaginitis, OTC products include antifungal agents such as clotrimazole, miconazole, econazole, and ketoconazole. You can also use plain old boric acid as a topical treatment for vaginal yeast infections and jock itch but NOT thrush. Boric acid is toxic if ingested. Ask your pharmacist to fill capsules with boric acid powder and follow directions for dosage and length of use.

According to former *Good Morning America* medical contributor Marie Savard, M.D., author most recently of *Ask Dr. Marie,* self-treating for yeast infections won't mask any other conditions. She also points out that topical OTC products cause no serious side effects. However, she cautions that creams and suppositories are typically oil based and therefore might weaken latex condoms and diaphragms.

Medical University of South Carolina researchers studying OTC treatment options for vaginitis found no significant differences among brands or formulations of any of the intravaginal imidazoles, a group of synthetic antifungal agents. However, they warned that vaginal anti-itch creams (including Vagisil, Vagi-gard, Summer's Eve, and Equate), which are often placed on shelves right next to vaginal yeast infection treatments, simply mask the symptoms and have no antifungal or antimicrobial effects. The active ingredients in these creams include benzocaine and resorcinol (for pain relief) as well as hydrocortisone (for itch relief). The researchers noted that women might gain only temporary relief or that the creams might actually worsen symptoms in some women. They pointed out that women with chronic yeast infections are not good candidates for OTC remedies and should see their doctors for prescription medications.

Be aware that, for both men and women, oral medications always pose a greater risk than creams because they pass through the liver. Dr. Marie is not a fan of oral medications for yeast vaginitis or jock itch, but she is aware that plenty of people prefer pills to creams, which can be messy. For patients who ask for oral meds, Dr. Marie prescribes fluconazole. It is marketed as Diflucan.

Oral thrush is fairly common in infants and can occur in adults as well. Babies usually get better with no treatment, but grown-ups can benefit from a prescription antifungal mouthwash such as nystatin or lozenges such as clotrimazole.

Antifungal Medications

When the time comes to start on antifungals after the 21-day Candida Cleanse, during Phase 2 of the diet, your doctor may prescribe one of the following FDA-approved medications.

Nystatin   This oral antifungal kills yeast by binding to a specific compound called ergosterol on the cell walls of the yeast, damaging it and causing potassium to leak, which results in the death of the cell. Nystatin effectively treats an overgrowth of Candida in the intestines, but it is not effective outside the digestive tract.

Oral amphotericin B   An antifungal with a structure very similar to that of nystatin, oral amphotericin B is effective in treating intestinal Candida overgrowth. Because the medication is not absorbed into the bloodstream, it does not cause unwanted side effects. Amphotericin B binds to the ergosterol on the cell wall of yeast, just as nystatin does.

Intravenous amphotericin   Acting throughout the body, this medication typically causes side effects including fever, chills, confusion, and anemia. However, these problems usually clear up within 12 hours. It is only called for when an infection is life-threatening.

Fluconazole   The oral antifungal fluconazole is safe and has minimal side effects. Its drawbacks are that it is very pricey and, unfortunately, Candida is developing a resistance to it.

Terbinafine HCL This medication is used either as an oral or topical treatment. (An OTC formulation is marketed for jock itch under the brand name Lamisil.) Terbinafine HCL has only mild side effects such as nausea and tummy aches, and so far Candida is not resistant to the drug.

Herbal Antifungal Supplements

Another possibility for treatment of Candida die-off is one of the herbal antifungals, which are available without a prescription. Again, these antifungals should be reserved for Phase 2 of the Candida Diet. Also, remember that herbs may interact with other drugs such as blood pressure medications, so be sure to let your doctor know if you are taking OTC supplements. Better yet, ask your pharmacist for help. He or she actually knows more about this subject than your doctor does.

Recent studies have shown that many herbal supplements, none of which are regulated by the FDA, may contain ingredients not listed on the labels and may in fact be dangerous. When Canadian researchers at the University of Guelph in Ontario looked at the DNA in 44 bottles of herbal products sold by 12 companies, they found that labeled ingredients often didn't reflect the actual contents. They used a test called DNA bar coding, which has been described as genetic fingerprinting. The scientists found that some products contained fillers, such as wheat or rice, not listed on the label. Some were contaminated with plant species that might cause allergic reactions, and others contained no trace at all of the herb supposedly in the bottle.

With that caution in mind, here's a list of the most popular herbal antifungals:

- **Pau d'arco tea**—Prepared from a South American herb widely recommended among alternative practitioners for Candida treatment.

- **Oregano oil**—Contains concentrated phenols, aromatic organic compounds that are purportedly effective in fighting bacterial infections, fungal infections, and Candida overgrowth.

- **Olive leaf extract**—Contains a substance that is said to fight Candida infections.

- **Neem**—Made from an evergreen native to India and used as an antifungal and detoxifier in Ayurvedic medicine.

- **Apple cider vinegar**—This is not actually an herb, but it needs to be on the list. It balances the pH level of the body and is thought to prevent Candida overgrowth.

- **Echinacea**—Most commonly used to fight the common cold but may also help with a person's immune reaction when fighting Candida.

- **Black walnut herbal supplement**—Contains tannins, water-soluble polyphenols that are reported to kill Candida overgrowth.

A Kansas State University microbiologist named Govindsamy Vediyappan, Ph.D., says he has found a breakthrough herbal medicine treatment for Candida overgrowth. He noticed that diabetic people in developing countries use a medicinal herb called *Gymnema sylvestre*—a tropical vine plant found in India, China, and Australia—to help control their sugar levels. He decided to study the microbiological use of the plant to learn whether it could beat back the Candida fungus. His research team purified gymnemic acid compounds in the plant leaves.

The team found that the gymnemic acid compounds purified from the plant leaves are nontoxic and that they block the invasive aspect of the fungus so the Candida becomes more treatable. The researchers also found that the compounds work quickly. Speed is an important characteristic because the treatable fungal yeast can jump to an out-of-control form with invasive branched filaments within 30 minutes of infection. At that stage, the filaments are hard to contain.

Dr. Vediyappan plans further research on the compounds and potential drug development. But until this type of promising new drug is available, I stick with my original advice: Get treatment for vaginal yeast infections, jock itch, and adult thrush right away, but hold off on other antifungals until you reach the "die-off" stage of the diet, typically after the 21-day cleanse but possibly earlier (or not at all).

Now, let's tackle a question that always comes up in connection with the topic of Candida overgrowth: Is a colonic necessary or even a good idea?

4

Do I Need a Colonic?

In a word, no. You may have heard that celebrities such as Kim Kardashian, Madonna, Leonardo DiCaprio, Halle Berry, Britney Spears, and Paris Hilton are big fans of colonics because the procedure purportedly gets rid of toxins and results in high-octane energy and less bloating. Well, get the stars out of your eyes. Colonic irrigation is not only expensive at well over $100 for just one visit, but also the process can be downright dangerous.

True, a colonic does loosen any hardened fecal matter in your intestines so that you quickly expel more Candida than you can get rid of by diet alone in the same amount of time. However, you'll also lose most of your good bacteria. Each colonic session, during which liquids are inserted into your rectum via a tube, lasts about 45 minutes. (A colonic is *not* the same as colonoscopy prep but is actually a cousin of the old-fashioned enema, a common home remedy for constipation years ago.)

Even advocates of colonics admit that the procedure can be stressful and exhausting. The typical recommendation is that you should plan to take several days off from work and cancel social activities so you can rest. Given all of that, and especially if you have any known health problems such as diabetes, steer clear of colonics and simply follow the Candida Cleanse diet. Your patience will pay off in the end.

A Risky Procedure

There are a number of risks in having a colonic. The procedure can cause perforations in your bowel. You may pick up bacterial infections from contaminated equipment. And flushing good, infection-fighting bacteria out of your gut can leave you vulnerable to infections.

Beyond that, a colonic can upset the balance of electrolytes in your system. Electrolytes are crucial for such functions as fluid absorption, regular heartbeats, and coordination of muscles. An imbalance of electrolytes can cause grave health problems, including heart attacks, seizures, and paralysis. Look at it this way: Electrolytes are salts that include sodium, potassium, chloride, bicarbonate, phosphate, calcium, and magnesium—all of which have key health functions.

Sodium: This regulates the amount of water in your body and is important for many body functions. Too much or too little sodium in your blood can be fatal.

Potassium: Potassium is vital for normal cells, regular heartbeats, and muscle function. An increase or decrease in potassium can negatively affect your nervous system and increase the risk of irregular heartbeats.

Chloride: Along with sodium, chloride helps your body maintain the correct balance of fluids.

Bicarbonate: This helps control the acidity of body fluids and blood. Upsetting the normal level of bicarbonate can affect respiratory and kidney functions.

Phosphate: Phosphate plays a part in the health of teeth and bones. It also helps with the utilization of carbohydrates and fats and is vital for the growth, maintenance, and repair of cells and tissues.

Calcium: Calcium makes teeth and bones strong and is essential for muscle contraction, nerve signaling, blood clotting, and heart function.

Magnesium: This is involved in over 300 biochemical reactions in the body, including muscle and nerve function, heart rhythm, immune system, bone strength, blood sugar levels, and normal blood pressure.

Given the importance of electrolytes, you can see why an imbalance caused by a colonic is extremely detrimental to your health. Yet another serious drawback of a colonic is that the herbal products used in many colonic treatments have been linked to various health problems such as liver toxicity and anemia. If you recall from the previous chapter, herbal products are not regulated and they are not always what they claim to be.

Home Colonic: A Very Bad Idea

If you decide you simply must have a colonic regardless of my advice, please never try a do-it-yourself colonic at home. You could end up rupturing your bowel wall and need surgery to repair it—if you're lucky. In 2003, the Texas attorney general filed lawsuits against colonic equipment manufacturers after a woman doing her own colonic irrigation ruptured her large intestine and died. The attorney general expressed this view: "We believe the routine use of these devices without a physician's approval or knowledge is like a ticking time bomb, and the patients may not be aware of the serious health risks involved." The lawsuits maintained that the use of colonic cleansing for "general well-being" and "re-energizing life" was fraudulent, and indeed that use is not approved by the FDA.

Beyond home equipment, there are many home products that claim to cleanse your colon, including Colovexus, Lipoclen, 7 Day Detox, 7 Day Colon Cleanser, and Colovox. None of them are cheap, but probably the most expensive cleanse is Gwyneth Paltrow's GOOP cleanse kit at over $400. Save your money. The Candida Cleanse diet is better for you, more effective, safer, and a whole lot less expensive!

If you still can't get colonics out of your mind, think about this: Long-term studies have found many reports of side effects, including cramping, bloating, nausea, vomiting, electrolyte imbalance, and impaired kidney function. And, please, definitely do not consider a colonic if you have an existing health condition such as Crohn's disease, ulcerative colitis, heart disease, kidney disease, diverticulitis, serious hemorrhoids, or cancer.

Be Safe

In spite of all the warnings from creditable sources against colonics, many websites and books about Candida overgrowth do sing their praises. I hope you'll ignore those testimonials and opt to proceed with the Candida Cleanse diet and forego a colonic. But if I have been unable to dissuade you from a colonic (seriously, think about it before you proceed), please heed these precautions:

- Consult your doctor first, especially if you have any health problems or take any prescription medicine.
- Be absolutely sure that the person performing the colonic will use disposable equipment that was not used before. Sterilizing isn't good enough—it should be brand new equipment that will be used just the one time.
- Some herbal supplements can cause health problems. Get a complete list of herbal ingredients

in any colon-cleansing products that will be used on you, and ask your pharmacist to look it over before you undergo the colonic.

• A colonic can easily dehydrate you and throw your electrolytes out of whack. Be sure to drink lots of fluids during and after colon cleansing.

I sincerely hope you'll avoid having a colonic—but if you do have one, please make sure the procedure is as safe as possible. Also, I want you to know that a colonic is not a cure for constipation and that you don't have to worry about becoming constipated on the Candida Cleanse diet. Read on to find out everything you need to know about "staying regular."

5

Constipation and Candida

Chronic constipation is a classic symptom of Candida overgrowth. The cleanse itself will relieve that problem in due time. However, if you need a little help while the diet is taking effect, Marie Savard, M.D., recommends a fiber supplement such as Metamucil, which is made from the husk of a plant whose common name is psyllium. She adds that osmotic laxatives such as Milk of Magnesia, stool softeners such as Ex-Lax, or glycerin suppositories can help.

Dr. Marie reminds us that these products don't have the phytonutrients and antioxidants found in high-fiber foods. Those foods are a mainstay of the Candida Cleanse diet, so the best advice is to stick with the regimen.

Why Constipation Is Harmful

Hard stools can cause straining, which in turn can cause hemorrhoids (varicose veins of the rectum). They may protrude and can bleed. If you're not "regular," with bowel movements every day or perhaps every other day, stool will remain in your colon for too long and become compacted. Incidentally, women have slower intestinal peristalsis—the contractions that move stools along—than men do. That's why women are so much more prone to constipation than men are.

Women are also more likely than men to have what Dr. Marie calls "safe toilet syndrome." That's when you hold it until you get home because you don't want to go in a strange place. The trouble is that by avoiding a movement, you are in effect creating constipation so that when you do get to your own bathroom, you either can't move your bowels or at least have difficulty with the process.

WHEN IT MAY BE MORE THAN CONSTIPATION

Simple constipation almost never requires a trip to the doctor. However, if you notice any of these possible signs of colon cancer, be sure to report them to your physician.

- Unexplained weight loss
- Change in your normal bowel habits
- Blood in your stool or the toilet other than from hemorrhoids

DON'T MAKE A PRACTICE OF HOLDING IT

If you put off heeding nature's call either because you're too busy or you don't want to use a bathroom while you're away from home, you are courting constipation. One woman in her 50s put it this way:

> I'm a first-grade teacher. There's no way I
> can leave the class alone in order to go to the
> bathroom. That means unless I have a bowel
> movement in the morning before I leave for school,
> I have to hold it until the lunch break. Then, by
> the time I get to the teachers' room to eat, I usually
> don't even feel as though I have to go any longer.
> Not only that, there are male teachers in the room
> and the bathroom is right off to one side so you
> can hear everything that goes on in there. I really
> hate the idea of pushing and making gassy noises
> and all the rest of it while the guys are listening.
>
> That's why I got into the habit of forcing myself
> to wait until I got home after school. I ended up so
> constipated that I was miserable. My solution was
> to start going home for lunch. Fortunately, I don't
> live very far from the school and once I started
> eating more fiber and drinking more water and
> giving myself a chance to use my own bathroom
> in private, I solved my problem. Eventually,
> once I was regular again, I almost always had my
> movement right after breakfast and then I went

back to eating lunch at school, which I had always enjoyed because of the camaraderie. All's well that ends well!

What Causes Constipation?

Candida overgrowth is a major cause of constipation, but so is a sedentary lifestyle, especially if you have a desk job. You need to stay physically active or else your entire system slows down, including your colon. Here's one woman's story:

> I was very active my whole life until I landed my first job after college as an administrative assistant at an advertising agency in New York City. I couldn't afford an apartment in the city, not even one with roommates, so I moved back in with my parents on Long Island. Yes, I was one of those boomerang kids, but what could I do? I kept telling myself that if I worked really hard and impressed my boss, I'd eventually get a raise and down the road I'd be promoted. The higher ups at the agency were making phenomenal salaries, especially the ones writing copy for pharmaceutical accounts. That's what I set my sights on while I was putting in 9 hours a day at the office with a 2-hour commute on either end on the Long Island Rail Road for a total of 4 hours a day. What that meant was that I had gone from being on the soccer team in college and training

for marathons to either sitting on a train or at my desk from dawn to dusk.

I promised myself I'd get some exercise on weekends but I was so drained by Friday night that all I wanted to do was sleep. The more sedentary I became, the more sluggish I felt. It was a vicious cycle. And before long, I was seriously constipated most of the time. Grabbing fast food to eat at my desk probably contributed to my condition, but it was the lack of activity that really did it. The reason I know that's true is that I finally confided in my mother about my, um, little problem. She made an appointment for me with the family doctor, and he said I had to start eating better but that the most important thing I could do was find a way to move more.

He recommended a software program that periodically disables your mouse and your keyboard so you're forced to take breaks. I started walking up and down the stairs of the office building during those breaks and I would also get up while I was on the train and walk up and down the aisle. People probably thought I was crazy but I didn't care. As for food, I started leaving the building and walking to a health food store during my lunch hour to get a turkey sandwich on whole grain bread with lettuce and tomato and no mayonnaise. For breakfast, I would have yogurt instead of a donut. My mom always did cook nutritious dinners, but I had been scarfing down ice cream after the meal. I stopped doing that. And guess what? Just those few changes in my daily routine gave me enough of my old energy back so that I was able to play soccer in an adult league on Saturday and Sunday. Before long, my constipation was cured. And, oh, I did get a raise and a promotion. Now I live in the city with my new boyfriend and I walk to and from work every day. I'll never let myself slip into a sedentary lifestyle again!

This woman's success story, of course, isn't simply about exercise. It's about eating well. Without even realizing it, she was following some of the basic tenets of the Candida Cleanse diet, and in fact it's a good bet she had Candida overgrowth because of the unhealthy lifestyle she was leading.

As she found out the hard way, one of the salient causes of constipation, a common symptom of Candida, is a diet without enough fiber to give you the bulk you need to move waste through your bowels. Dr. Marie describes the colon as "a muscle that needs a daily workout." Fiber stretches the muscle. Then after a bowel movement, the muscle goes back to its original state. However, chronic constipation can stretch the colon too much. When that happens, the muscle loses its natural elasticity and no longer springs back effectively.

Drinking too few fluids can also cause constipation. You need about 1½ to 2 quarts a day. Water is best, but all fluids count. Keep in mind that sugary drinks are absolutely verboten on the Candida Cleanse. Beyond that, see Chapter 11 for advice about coffee, artificial sweeteners, and alcohol. And here's a surprising fact: Although tea is generally good for you, it can actually slow down peristalsis.

Other Reasons for Constipation

In addition to the most significant causes of constipation—poor diet and a sedentary lifestyle—here are a few less common ones:

- "Holiday constipation," when the hustle and bustle plus festive food and drink can upset your routine and cause you to stray from your healthy eating and lifestyle habits
- Travel that involves sitting for long periods on planes and trains or in cars
- Pregnancy, when the extra weight and a rise in the levels of the hormone progesterone can slow down peristalsis
- Uterine fibroids, especially if they are large
- Prescription medications, including antidepressants, opioids, diuretics, and some calcium channel blockers

- Over-the-counter medicines such as antihistamines, cough medicines, and iron tablets
- An underactive thyroid gland
- Diabetes
- Multiple sclerosis
- Depression
- Diverticulitis

The key to conquering constipation is to stick faithfully to the Candida Cleanse while also paying attention to any factors contributing to your problem. A combination of eating to beat back the fungus and making positive lifestyle changes will get you regular again. However, don't heed the siren call of an "all-liquid cleanse" to solve constipation. Read on to find out why.

6

Is an All-Liquid Cleanse Necessary?

If you've done any searching on the Internet in your quest to fight Candida overgrowth, you have surely stumbled on various sites that advocate all-liquid cleanses. Don't be fooled! An all-liquid cleanse is not only unnecessary but also bad for you in several ways.

Risks of an All-Liquid Cleanse

First of all, a liquid diet does not promote the good muscle tone you need if your colon is to function as it should. Subsisting on liquids alone practically guarantees that you'll end up constipated—and that you'll probably further upset the balance of the microorganisms in your gut. You'll get better and longer lasting results if your cleanse includes fiber-rich foods such as low-carbohydrate vegetables.

FORGET THE MASTER CLEANSE

The most highly touted liquid cleanse, called the Master Cleanse or the Lemonade Diet, is the one made famous when the pop star Beyoncé recommended it during an appearance she made on *The Oprah Winfrey Show* in 2006. The Master Cleanse consists of a drink made of water, lemon juice, maple syrup or molasses, and cayenne pepper that you consume six or more times a day. Since a major component of the Candida Cleanse is eliminating sugar in order to starve the fungus, the sugar content of the drink is obviously at odds with that goal. There's no way that the standard Lemonade Diet, with its heavy reliance on sugar in the form of maple syrup or molasses, will help you beat back Candida. In fact, if you didn't already have Candida overgrowth when you started that diet, you probably would by the time you drank your last glass of the lemonade!

The Master Cleanse dates back to the 1940s, when Stanley Burroughs, who philosophized on and wrote about health and diet, introduced it as a detoxification method meant to last from 4 to 14 days. It experienced a resurgence after Beyoncé claimed to have lost 20 pounds on the cleanse. Other celebrities, including Ashton Kutcher and Demi Moore, jumped on the bandwagon, fans followed suit, and social media lit up with testimonials to the wonders of the Master Cleanse, which supposedly not only helped people pare off pounds but also cured acne and made the believers feel strong and energetic. If those claims are tempting you to give the liquid cleanse a try, get a grip and remind yourself that the Candida Cleanse diet with its emphasis on vegetables, fiber, and real food safely does all of that and much more.

After the liquid cleanse gained a lot of public attention, nutritionists and health experts began to speak out against it. They criticized the fact that it depletes the body of essential nutrients and pointed out that any weight loss was fleeting. In fact, Beyoncé has since gone on record saying that she gave up the liquid cleanse and now eats a healthy diet and exercises more.

Maybe you've heard that there is a version of the Master Cleanse using artificially sweetened maple syrup. But watch out! Artificial sweeteners are of questionable value and may even be harmful; see Chapter 11 for more information.

You should know that unsweetened lemon juice itself is allowed on the Candida Cleanse diet. The juice of lemons and limes changes the acid-alkaline balance in the body for the better. The juice is acidic, but it ramps up digestive secretions that alkalize your system and helps in the fight against Candida overgrowth. As you'll see when we get to the diet itself, there are many ways to include unsweetened lemon juice in your diet, such as squeezing it on fish and vegetables or using it to make a salad dressing.

BEWARE BENTONITE

Yet another version of the all-liquid cleanse involves vegetable broth and a drink made from a form of clay called bentonite. It can be very dangerous, especially for pregnant women and the elderly. Also, why cook vegetables to make a broth and then throw away the vegetables, which are such terrific sources of fiber? Again, an all-liquid cleanse, no matter which version you're considering, is not a good idea.

Quick Fix vs. Eating for Life

Another reason not to submit yourself to an all-liquid cleanse is that you won't be re-educating yourself by forming new, healthy eating habits as you will on the Candida Cleanse diet. Phase 1 of the diet will give you amazing results in just 21 days, and then you'll move on to Phases 2 and 3, during which you'll learn to enjoy nutritious food for the rest of your life. One woman who tried an all-liquid cleanse had the following experience:

> I'll admit I was looking for a quick fix when it came to losing weight and clearing my Candida symptoms. This was back in 2007 when the Lemonade Diet was all the rage. I figured if it was good enough for Beyoncé and Demi Moore, it was good enough for me. I've always wanted a body like the celebrities on the red carpet at award shows and I decided this was the way to lose my midlife muffin top. Also, I had been feeling spacey

and having other Candida symptoms so I figured the Lemonade cleanse would kill two birds with one stone.

Well, I stuck with the cleanse for the full 2 weeks, and I did lose 10 pounds. But I felt awful! I'd read these tweets from people saying the cleanse gave them a lot of pep and I was mystified. Maybe they didn't have Candida. For me, the maple sugar was exactly what I didn't need! I figured that out after I learned more about what a healthy Candida Cleanse diet is all about.

I had never had very good eating habits, but eating to beat back the fungus taught me a whole new approach to nutrition. My friends couldn't believe it! My nickname used to be Sugar Mama because I had the worst sweet tooth in history. I was practically keeping Dunkin' Donuts and Entenmann's in business. I hardly ever ate veggies. All of that changed. I know I can't go back to my old ways even for a little while. But why would I want to do that? I feel younger than I have in years, my skin is clear, I wake up full of energy, and I'm never in a fog. I thought I was having senior moments even though I'm only in my 40s, but it was just that the overgrowth was doing me in. Now I tell everyone about eating right to conquer the fungus. Honestly, I think anybody would feel better on this diet whether they had overgrowth or not. As for the liquid cleanse, never again!

I hope that by now you're convinced that an all-liquid cleanse is a stopgap at best and a health risk at worst. Even so, I realize that one reason the liquid diet seems so appealing is that there is the promise of weight loss. Never fear! As you'll learn in Chapter 9, the healthy Candida Cleanse diet can help you lose weight effectively and safely at a pace that will keep you from diet rebound, the phenomenon of regaining every ounce you lost.

But I know what you're thinking. Does the Candida Cleanse diet really beat back the fungus. The next chapter gives you the answer!

7

Does the Candida Cleanse Diet Really Work?

Yes! The Candida Cleanse can work even for people who previously ate the worst possible diets. Here's the firsthand experience of a woman who had no idea what healthy eating was like before embarking on a diet to beat back Candida:

> I'm a Boomer who grew up in the 1950s on a diet of Campbell's soup, meatloaf, potato chips, french fries, 3 Musketeers, Nesbitt's orange soda, Reddi-wip, creamed chipped beef on toast, grilled Velveeta sandwiches on Wonder Bread, peanut butter and jelly sandwiches on Wonder Bread, lots of milk, plenty of ice cream, and a Fig Newton in each hand when I went to bed. Add to that the holiday meals with pickles, stuffing, candied yams, pies, cake, and all the rest and you can see that I was eating a totally unhealthy diet.

My parents and all their friends drank cocktails and smoked, which I thought was very grown up and glamorous, so I took up those habits as soon as I was old enough. My mother's favorite drink was a Manhattan made with whiskey, sweet vermouth, and bitters. That's the one that I decided to drink every evening as well—sometimes two of them, to be honest. And I kept on eating the way I did as a kid. I would actually crumble potato chips into my Campbell's tomato soup! Oh, I forgot. I also put ketchup on just about everything except dessert!

By the time I was in my late 20s, I felt ancient. I could barely get out of bed and the fatigue dogged me all day. Plus, I had a job as a receptionist in a law firm so I was getting no exercise at all. I would skip breakfast, eat a fast-food lunch at my desk, go home to have my Manhattan, and order pizza or make Hamburger Helper plus a baked potato with plenty of sour cream and butter. Then I would fall into bed, but I usually didn't sleep very well and I often woke up feeling sick to my stomach.

Finally, I went to my doctor and she was actually the one who recommended what amounted to an anti-Candida diet, although she didn't call it that. She put me on a strict, healthy regimen without sugar or white flour and with plenty of vegetables and some fruit. She also told me to quit drinking and smoking. Well, believe it or not, I decided to make all three of those big lifestyle changes at the same time and I succeeded! My parents had both died fairly young of heart attacks so I guess my motivation was the desire to live long and live healthy. Little did I know that I was not only beginning to be heart healthy but that I was also beating back Candida overgrowth. I had been getting vaginal yeast infections off and on for years but I never made the connection to the way I was eating. Anyway, when I started feeling better, I went to the library to do some research. This was before Google! So, there I was at the card catalogue and I stumbled on information about *Candida albicans.* I asked my doctor about antifungals. That turned out to be the missing piece I needed.

All I can say is that anybody who tells you the diet doesn't work is probably not sticking with it. You can't go back to the way you used to eat and expect to stay well and then blame the diet! The diet worked, or I should say works, for me. I brought up my two children to eat well and I also retrained my husband. Now I'm a grandmother and I'm proud to say that my kids are great parents who have taught their kids to eat a healthy diet. I don't think they'll ever get overgrowth in the first place.

This woman whose story you just read no doubt hit on the real reason some experts and sufferers alike say the diet doesn't work: recidivism. That's a fancy word for a tendency to relapse into a previous mode of behavior. Fortunately, though, the Candida Diet is easy to stick to because it's so sensible and offers a lot of food choices. Even if you've tried diets in the past and failed, you'll find that the Candida Diet isn't about deprivation. It's a completely different approach to eating that is not only satisfying but will make you healthier, in the same way that it did for the woman whose story you just read. That's great motivation to follow the diet faithfully. If you also get the antifungals you need during Phase 2, I know you'll become a believer!

Even so, you may be wondering if the diet is not only effective but also safe. The next chapter tackles that issue.

8

Is the Candida Diet Safe?

The answer is "yes." You will eat real food rather than processed products. You will eliminate or greatly reduce your
intake of unhealthy items, including sugar and white flour.
You will almost certainly consume more vegetables, which
are great sources of good carbohydrates. All of these factors mean that the diet is very beneficial for you and not
risky at all as long as you follow it thoughtfully.

Don't Go to Extremes

The danger lies in taking the advice in this book to
extremes. Here's how one person did exactly that:

> I wanted to try an anti-Candida diet for two
> reasons: I was getting a lot of infections, including
> vaginal yeast and athlete's foot and I also wanted
> to slim down. I couldn't zip my favorite jeans any
> longer and I was gaining more weight every month
> even though I wasn't eating all that differently than
> I had been before I hit menopause. I guess your

metabolism just slows down as you get older. Well, I wasn't about to give in to that so I started the diet.

I felt better almost immediately and I didn't really have die-off relapse. I was also losing about a pound a week. This was all very encouraging so I decided to see if I could lose even more weight. My high school reunion was coming up in a couple of months and I wanted to look good. I cut out all meat and eggs and ate only the permitted vegetables. To be honest, since I was seeing great results on the scale, I think I kind of slipped into an eating disorder.

My husband was getting very concerned, but I told him he shouldn't worry and that I was fine. Then I got to the point where just the thought of eating anything but a salad terrified me. I envisioned gaining back everything I had lost and then some. Finally, my husband insisted that I go to my doctor and she talked some sense into me. End of story, no diet is "safe" if you take it to extremes. Don't mess with what an anti-Candida diet is all about. You're playing Russian roulette with your health if you do!

Healthy Diet Equals Healthy Aging

A healthy way of eating increases your chances of healthy aging. Let me tell you about some research showing the association between dietary patterns at midlife and health as we age. The research was done as part of the Nurses' Health Study, one of the largest and longest running studies on women's health. Between 1984 and 1986, the researchers looked at the diets of 10,670 women with no major chronic diseases when they were in their late 50s and early 60s. Then they had the women provide information on their health an average of 15 years later.

The diet the healthy women followed was a version of the Mediterranean diet, which is very similar to the Candida Cleanse diet except that it allows more fruit and some other foods that aren't permitted on the Candida Cleanse, such as peanuts and cow's milk dairy products (except for yogurt). What can we conclude from the research? Following a Mediterranean-style diet, which avoids sugar, white flour, and processed foods, seems to substantially boost the chances for a healthy old age.

Here are the major dos and don'ts of the Mediterranean diet. They can easily be applied to the Candida Cleanse diet as well.

- **Fruits and Vegetables**—These "good carbohydrates," whether fresh, canned, or cooked, are nutrition powerhouses. They also have fiber that helps prevent constipation.
- **Whole Grains**—A variety of whole grains that have not been stripped of the husks containing essential

B vitamins and fiber are strongly recommended in lieu of the less nutritious "white" versions.

- **Nuts and Seeds**—These are ideal as snacks because they have fiber, protein, and fats that are good for you.

- **Healthy Oils**—Olive oil is ideal. Other oils such as coconut and sesame are fine but aren't used as often in the Mediterranean countries. Substitute the oils for butter or margarine, which have unhealthy fats.

- **Spices and Herbs**—Skip the salt. Instead, make food more tempting by cooking with a wide range of these flavor- and aroma-enhancers that won't raise blood pressure.

- **Fish**—Breading and frying aren't allowed but eating broiled or baked fresh fish twice a week or more supplies heart-healthy omega3 fatty acids plus lean protein. Water-packed fish is also an option.

- **Red Meat in Moderation**—Have beef only about once a month. Choose lean cuts and have small portions.

- **No High-Fat Processed Meats**—Stay away from sausages, whether fresh or smoked, because they all contain salt and sugar. Also avoid bacon, salami, pepperoni, bologna, bratwurst, and hot dogs.

Is This Diet Safe for My Kids?

Yes, although you should ask your pediatrician whether you need to start the children at Phase 2, especially if they have no Candida overgrowth symptoms and you simply want them to learn to eat healthy foods. You'll be doing them a favor if you get them to cut out sweets and white flour and to stop eating processed and fast foods. Here is one mother's story:

> I'll admit I used to let my kids have plenty of candy and desserts. My son was a picky eater, and I found I could coax him into having at least some vegetables if I promised him a treat or ice cream as a reward. My daughter was better about eating whatever I served her, but of course she would get jealous if I didn't give her candy or ice cream when I gave some to her brother. By the time Jason was five and Caroline was three, the pediatrician said that they were overweight. I just thought they were chubby and cute, but the doctor was very stern with me. For that matter, so was the dentist. Both kids already had some cavities.
>
> Right about that time, my cousin told me about her battle with Candida overgrowth. Something just clicked when I heard her list of symptoms. I was experiencing a lot of them myself! I cut out sugar and white flour, and I got my husband to do that as well. Before long we were feeling better, so

that's when I realized I had to stop giving in to my kids when it came to treats and desserts. I started leaving the kids with my husband when I went to the grocery store so they wouldn't whine and fuss about wanting me to buy candy and ice cream. I just toughed it out even though my son wasn't eating enough vegetables without the promise of a reward.

Long story short, my son finally came around. I still allow treats on birthdays and holidays, but we make a ritual of throwing out any leftover cake and ice cream and other goodies the next day. By now my children are in middle school, and they are both at a healthy weight and very active in sports. I credit my new way of eating to beat back the fungus with setting my kids on a lifelong path to a healthy lifestyle.

Is This Diet Safe for Older People?

Yes, again! Recent research has shown that inflammation may be the primary cause of aging and many age-related diseases. Follow the Candida Cleanse diet and you'll stand a very good chance of feeling younger than your years as you age. Also, if you are a caregiver, you will be maintaining the health and strength you need in order to do well by your loved one. You might even want to help the person in your charge to begin eating better and exercising as well. This is how one woman did exactly that:

> My mother was 89 when she came to live with us. She was very frail but thank goodness she still had all of her faculties. I was eating to beat back the fungus and so we started preparing meals together. We made snack bags of broccoli, carrots, and cauliflower and we experimented with herbs and spices. The time we spent together in the kitchen reminded both of us of the times when my brother and I were little and my mom would let us cook with her even if we made a mess. It was great for us to bond like that again!

> Also, I read somewhere that if the frail elderly sit in a chair and lift ankle weights, they will gain strength. I bought some weights and my mom was really good about doing the exercises. I'd do them with her and we put music on to make it more fun. Then I bought some resistance bands and we added to our exercise routine. Before long, Mom was walking much better and we both felt better!

That's certainly inspiring. As always, remember to see your doctor before embarking on any diet or exercise program. And that goes double if you and yours are 50 or older.

Now, let's move on to the next chapter where you'll learn how the Candida Cleanse diet can be a weight loss diet if you need to pare off pounds.

9

The Candida Cleanse and Weight Loss

Most people do lose weight on the first phase, the 21-day Candida Cleanse, simply because the typical overgrowth sufferer previously ate calorie-laden foods containing sugar and white flour. Switching to a low-sugar, low-carbohydrate regimen with an emphasis on vegetables and high-quality protein should definitely help get rid of any excess pounds.

As you've surely heard by now, there's an obesity epidemic in America and even people who don't qualify as obese may be having trouble maintaining a healthy weight. If you're among that number, then the Candida Cleanse will almost certainly deliver a one-two punch for you by starving the fungus and slimming you down at the same time.

Body Mass Index

One way to figure out whether you're carrying a healthy amount of weight is to figure out your body mass index, or BMI.

The National Heart, Lung, and Blood Institute puts it plainly: The higher your BMI, the higher your risk for heart disease, high blood pressure, type 2 diabetes, gallstones, breathing problems, and some cancers, including colon cancer. Note, however, that BMI may overestimate body fat in athletes and others who have a muscular build and it may underestimate body fat in older people and others who have lost muscle.

You can find BMI calculators on the Internet or you can figure out your BMI with this simple formula: BMI = $703 \times$ weight (in pounds) $\div$ height (in inches). These are the BMI categories:

Underweight	Below 18.5
Normal	18.5–24.9
Overweight	25.0–29.9
Obesity	30.0 and above

Waist Circumference and Waist-to-Hip Ratio

Another key to finding out if you're at a healthy weight is to measure the circumference of your waist. Because belly fat (white fat), as opposed to good fat (brown fat), is blamed for many diseases, some experts now say that a higher than recommended waist measurement is the most important indicator of the need to lose weight.

The National Institutes of Health reports that if most of your fat is around your waist rather than at your hips, you're at an increased risk for heart disease and type 2 diabetes. This risk goes up with a waist size that is greater than 35 inches for women or greater than 40 inches for men. The NIH gives these directions for correctly measuring your waist: Stand and place a tape measure around your middle, just above your hip bones. Measure your waist just after you breathe out.

Marie Savard, M.D., gives an even more detailed explanation in her book *Ask Dr. Marie,* but she isn't satisfied with just a waist measurement. She firmly believes that you need to know your waist-to-hip ratio, or WHR.

Start with the waist. Dr. Marie advises measuring at the narrowest point, where your waistband or a belt would go. Another guideline is to find the bottom of your rib cage. She notes that many sources, including the Centers for Disease Control and Prevention, suggest measuring around the area where your belly button is. However, as an expert on WHR, Dr. Marie says the resulting number from measuring your waist that way is not accurate, especially for women.

She also warns that you shouldn't cheat yourself out of a true measurement by sucking in your gut or pulling the tape measure tight enough to indent your flesh. "The idea is to face once and for all exactly how many inches around your abdomen really is," she says. "Nobody has to know this information except you! Seriously, not even your doctor is likely to find out. The value of WHR is well known by physicians but the majority of them still don't whip out a tape measure during your annual physical and keep track of the results year by year. They continue to rely on your weight and height although those numbers fall far short of your WHR as a health indicator."

Next, measure your hips at the widest place. Then divide your waist measurement by your hip measurement. Here are the cutoffs for healthy results: a waist size of 35 inches or less for women and 40 or less for men, and a WHR of 8 or less.

Calorie Counting

If your BMI and WHR results indicate that you ought to lose weight, you can make the Candida Cleanse diet work even better for you by paying attention to the calories in the foods you eat and to calories burned from exercise. There are 3,500 calories in 1 pound of body fat. That means, to lose 1 pound you need a deficit of 3,500 calories. Starting with that number, you can figure out how much weight you can lose through exercise or cutting calories, or both. Here are some examples:

- Walking or jogging uses approximately 100 calories per mile. You will lose 1 pound for every

35 miles walked, as long as your calorie intake and exercise remain constant.

- Walking briskly at a pace of 4 miles per hour for 30 minutes on 5 out of 7 days adds up to 10 miles a week. It will take you 3½ weeks to lose 1 pound if your calorie intake stays the same.

- If you reduce your food intake by 250 calories a day, you will lose 1 pound in 2 weeks even without exercising.

However, exercise plus fewer calories is the best way to slim down more quickly. By eating 250 fewer calories a day and walking briskly for 30 minutes a day for 8 days, you will lose 1 pound in just over a week. Reducing calorie intake even more and exercising more will speed up the process significantly.

If You Don't Need to Lose Weight

For most people, BMI and WHR measurements indicate that at least a little if not a lot of weight loss on the Candida Cleanse diet is beneficial. However, if you're already at your ideal weight or below, you should make certain to consume enough calories so you don't get too thin. Your best bet is to increase your intake of the following allowed foods:

- Fish—A 3-ounce serving of salmon contains just 121 calories, but you could double that amount for a 6-ounce serving.

- **Chicken**—A 3-ounce breast without skin has only about 140 calories, but with skin the calorie count is more like 190. Again, try having larger portions and do eat the skin.

- **Avocado**—One cup of sliced avocado has 234 calories. Increase the number of times a week you have this permitted food.

- **Eggs**—A large egg has only 70 calories. Although you don't want to eat too many of them each week, you should be able have four to six with no problem.

- **Nuts**—One almond contains 7 calories. So go ahead and enjoy a handful or two fairly often. The same applies to other nuts on the permitted list (see page 123).

- **Olive oil**—Like many other oils, 1 tablespoon of olive oil has 120 calories—but this is an especially healthy fat. Use it liberally as a salad dressing, in cooking, and to dribble on entrées.

- **Beef**—Most cuts as well as ground beef have about 190 calories for a 3-ounce serving. As with eggs, you don't want to overindulge, but eating somewhat more beef should be fine. As always, check with your doctor.

Next, let's learn about an essential part of the Candida Cleanse: prebiotics and probiotics.

10

The Importance of Prebiotics and Probiotics

Both prebiotics and probiotics are essential in the Candida Cleanse diet. Prebiotics are indigestible carbohydrates that act as food for probiotics, which contain live bacteria. Together, they help promote the growth of the good bacteria in your intestines and maintain your gut's ecosystem. When a food contains both substances, it is called synbiotic: a synergistic combination of the two.

Prebiotics

A form of dietary fiber, prebiotics occur naturally in plants, although in tiny amounts. They are resistant to heat from cooking and to stomach acid, and they cannot be digested. They move through the digestive system to the large intestine, where they nourish beneficial gut bacteria.

There's no need for prebiotic supplements because you'll almost certainly get all the prebiotics you need from the Candida Cleanse diet. In Phases 2 and 3, however, you could look for cereal and bread with prebiotics added. Onions and garlic are terrific sources of prebiotics, so use them liberally. Eat plenty of asparagus, artichokes, dandelion greens, leeks, and chicory. You could also buy roasted chicory root to use as a coffee substitute.

Probiotics

These beneficial bacteria that colonize the gastrointestinal tract are essential for good health. The research conducted thus far about the role of probiotics is encouraging. It indicates that probiotics do the following:

- Help stop diarrhea, including bouts that happen as a result of taking antibiotics.
- Stave off vaginal yeast infections and urinary tract infections, and help treat those that may occur anyway.
- Ease the symptoms of irritable bowel syndrome.
- Lower the risk of bladder cancer recurring.
- Help with healing intestinal infections more quickly.
- Ward off eczema and aid in curing established cases of the condition.

- Reduce the likelihood of contracting colds and flu, and make the illnesses less severe if they do happen.

Here are some good sources of probiotics:

YOGURT

Look for the words "live active cultures" on the label—that tells you the yogurt is a source of probiotics. Yogurt is considered synbiotic because it contains both the bacteria and the fuel the bacteria need to thrive.

In addition to all the reasons I just listed that probiotics are good for you, yogurt turns out to have an additional benefit. A University of California, Los Angeles study of women who regularly consumed yogurt with probiotics provides the first evidence that changing the bacterial environment, or microbiota, in the gut can positively affect brain function.

The lead researcher, Karen Tillisch, M.D., noted that many people eat yogurt because they like it or for the calcium content, but the study findings indicate yogurt may do much more than that—it may change the way a person's brain responds to the environment. In fact, just 4 weeks of yogurt-with-probiotics consumption was enough to show a difference in the activity of brain regions that control central processing of emotion and sensation.

Most probiotic products have never been studied. Dr. Tillisch pointed out that these products contain different strains of bacteria. As for whether or not different people need different strains, or whether some strains are more beneficial, the jury is out until more research is done. She did observe that some studies have shown that people with irritable bowel syndrome do better when they eat yogurt containing probiotics.

That observation brings us back from the fascinating research on yogurt and the brain to the effect of yogurt on your gut microbiota. The probiotics in yogurt help balance your intestinal system by restoring your supply of good bacteria, which was depleted by Candida overgrowth. Probiotics are thought to keep Candida from growing any further because of antifungal substances that the good bacteria release. They also give off lactic and acetic acids, which keep your gut acidic, the way it should be.

KEFIR

Kefir (pronounced kee-fur) is a fermented probiotic drink made by mixing milk—preferably goat, sheep, or coconut milk—with a starter usually referred to as "kefir grains." The drink is thought to have originated in the northern Caucasus Mountains around 3,000 B.C. You can easily make kefir at home. Kefir starter kits, which are sold online, typically only last for five to seven uses. However, if you buy the grains themselves instead, which are also available online at Amazon and other sites, you will have more and more grains left each time you create a batch, and you can reuse the grains indefinitely. Each batch takes about 24 to 48 hours to ripen.

SAUERKRAUT

Sauerkraut, which is German for "sour cabbage," is fermented with the probiotic bacteria leuconostoc, pediococcus, and lactobacillus. Warning: Don't buy the pasteurized sauerkraut sold in most supermarkets. The process of pasteurization kills the beneficial bacteria. Do an online Google search for "unpasteurized sauerkraut" instead.

KIMCHI

This is the national dish of Korea. It is made by fermenting vegetables such as cabbage, radishes, scallions, and cucumbers. The flavor is both spicy and sour.

There are many varieties and all of them not only have probiotics but are also good sources of vitamins.

MISO

The Japanese have this fermented soybean paste for breakfast and it's also often made into a soup. Miso has more than 160 strains of probiotic bacteria.

TEMPEH

Another probiotic food made from fermented soybeans, this one is a high-protein Indonesian patty that has a natural antibiotic. The flavor is not unlike that of a mushroom. The patty can be a substitute for red meat.

PROBIOTIC CAPSULES AND POWDER

You could take one of the many probiotic over-the-counter supplements available in either capsule or powder form. They are equally effective. Taking the supplements with food helps with efficient delivery of the bacteria. As always, check with your doctor and pharmacist before taking any supplement.

Read labels carefully since the various products contain differing amounts of bacteria. You're better off starting with a low amount and increasing it gradually, staying alert for Candida die-off, and cutting back temporarily if that happens. (See Chapter 22 to learn more about die-off.)

Some probiotic products contain just one strain of bacteria while others have as many as 15 or more. Whether the extra strains are beneficial is open to question, but the most powerful strains are generally regarded to be *Lactobacillus acidophilus* and *Bifidobacterium bifidum*. L. acidophilus reportedly boosts your immune system and helps beat back Candida overgrowth. L. acidophilus DDS-1 is an even more powerful cousin of this strain. B. bifidum is supposed to aid digestion, keep your immune system functioning well, and help synthesize B vitamins.

Certain probiotic supplements also contain prebiotics. However, you should get enough prebiotics simply by following the 21-day Candida Cleanse and the subsequent phases of the diet.

As I mentioned earlier in this chapter, you can enjoy roasted chicory root—a coffee substitute—as a source of prebiotics. Speaking of coffee, the next chapter deals with the question of whether or not caffeine is okay on the Candida Cleanse. I'll also discuss whether gluten, alcohol, and artificial sweeteners are permissible.

11

What About Gluten, Caffeine, Alcohol, and Artificial Sweeteners?

During the initial 21 days of the Candida Cleanse, gluten, caffeine, alcohol, and artificial sweeteners are not allowed. When you reach Phase 2, you can start experimenting with all of them except gluten, which you shouldn't try until Phase 3.

Here's what you need to know about each of those substances:

Gluten

A mixture of proteins in cereal grains, especially wheat, gluten is often blamed for a long list of health ills—and Candida is sometimes accused of triggering a sensitivity to gluten. Many people claim they are allergic to gluten, but the fact is that a true gluten allergy, as in celiac disease, is rare. That said, people who stop eating wheat and switch to other grains such as corn and rye typically say they feel much better.

Grains are not allowed on the initial 21-day Candida Cleanse, and to err on the side of caution, wheat and wheat products are not permitted during Phase 2. If you really want to test your tolerance for gluten, you can reintroduce wheat during Phase 3, at least occasionally. However, should your symptoms return, you should eliminate wheat again.

Caffeine

You need to eliminate coffee, colas, black tea, and other sources of caffeine during the 21-day Candida Cleanse. Decaf coffee still has some caffeine, so avoid decaf as well. Green tea is allowed. Then during Phases 2 and 3, you can test whether or not you can tolerate caffeine, especially in coffee. Keep in mind that caffeine in the late afternoon and early evening can disrupt sleep at night. Researchers at the American Academy of Sleep Medicine recently proved that caffeine even 6 hours before bedtime can significantly interfere with sleep.

Other studies have found health benefits associated with drinking coffee. Jana Klauer, M.D., author of *The Park Avenue Nutritionist's Plan,* is an enthusiastic proponent of coffee, which she points out contains healthful compounds. In fact, she asserts that because we drink so much coffee, it's the primary source of antioxidants in the American diet.

Dr. Klauer notes that two large studies show that drinking coffee lowers the risk of type 2 diabetes. She also points to a study indicating that long-term coffee drinking may protect against cognitive decline and Alzheimer's disease. According to the study, the polyphenol compounds in coffee triggered the release of an anti-inflammatory protein that increased nerve growth and improved nerve transmission in the brain.

Other benefits of coffee consumption that Dr. Klauer cites are prostate cancer prevention and weight loss. As for caffeine, she maintains that it increases alertness and reaction speed because it blocks adenosine, a chemical in the body that acts as a natural sleeping pill. Finally, she points to caffeine's pain-relieving properties. Yet she cautions that moderation is the key and notes that you should not drink coffee if you have cardiac arrhythmia (irregular heartbeat) or are pregnant.

An Italian study found that coffee consumption reduces the risk of liver cancer. The American Gastroenterological Association notes that the main causes of liver cancer are chronic hepatitis infections but that other risk factors include diabetes and obesity. Coffee has been proven to curb type 2 diabetes, obviously another fact in its favor. (I have to point out that the Candida Cleanse diet itself, because it's so healthy and cuts out sugar, is a great way to keep diabetes and obesity at bay!)

Although I wouldn't heed the advice of some Candida Diet advocates to avoid coffee altogether, in the end the decision is up to you. See for yourself how you react to coffee during Phases 2 and 3. If you can tolerate it, fine. If not, eliminate it.

Artificial Sweeteners

Researchers at Yale University found that the brain isn't fooled by fake sugar. In fact, artificial sweeteners could lead to sugar consumption later because our pleasure in eating sweets is largely driven by the amount of energy it provides rather than by the flavor. That means zero-calorie diet drinks now could lead to full-calorie versions later, after the low-cal drinks fail to satisfy.

Because eliminating sugar to starve the fungus is a key component of the Candida Cleanse, it's important to use artificial sweeteners sparingly and not until Phases 2 and 3. Even then, avoid aspartame and sucralose since they can raise your blood glucose just as sugar does—and that's exactly what the fungus wants. Also, aspartame may be carcinogenic. Brand names for aspartame and sucralose include NutraSweet, Equal, Spoonful, and Equal-Measure.

When you do choose to use a sweetener, your best bet is the natural sweetener stevia. It's made from the leaves of a plant popularly known as sweetleaf or sugarleaf rather than being manufactured in a lab, and it has almost no carbohydrates. Also, it does not spike your blood glucose. Look for a brand called Better Stevia. Some other brands have dextrose or other sweeteners that you should avoid. Be aware, however, that stevia has an unpleasant aftertaste—so much so that many users give up on this option.

Another possibility is xylitol, which can be called a natural sweetener when it is extracted from plant sources such as berries, oats, and mushrooms, as well as from the fibrous material of corn husks and birch. However, xylitol is also industrially produced, and in those instances it is synthetic or artificial. Dentists actually recommend gum with xylitol because it helps prevent cavities. Some brands of xylitol that you can use occasionally in your Phase 2 or 3 meal plans are Xlear XyloSweet, Health Garden Kosher Birch Xylitol, and Emerald Forest. Xylitol doesn't increase your blood glucose and is therefore included in foods designed for diabetics. Warning: Xylitol can be poisonous for your pets so keep it out of their reach and call your vet immediately if Fido or Fluffy manages to swallow some!

Alcohol

Alcoholic drinks are off limits during the 21-day Candida Cleanse because all of them except hard liquor contain at least some sugar and most people drink hard liquor in cocktails rather than "neat." You could probably get away with a shot or two of hard liquor during the cleanse, but don't forget that drinking can weaken your self-control and your resolve to stick with the diet.

The late William G. Crook, M.D., author of *The Yeast Connection: A Medical Breakthrough* first published in the mid-1980s, maintained that because wines and beers contain yeast, you should not include them in your diet. That is faulty reasoning since although *Candida albicans* is a yeast, it doesn't feed on yeast. Even so, the carbohydrates in wine and beer do feed the fungus. You can go ahead and experiment with having an occasional drink when you get to Phase 2 or 3 but if your symptoms come back, you'll need to stop imbibing.

Onward now to the question of whether or not organic foods—almost always pricey—are better than the rest of what's available in your supermarket.

12

Organic Foods: Are They Safer and More Nutritious?

Organic foods are harvested or produced from crops grown without synthetic pesticides, chemical fertilizers, industrial solvents, radiation, or chemical food additives. Organic meats and poultry are from free-range animals raised on organic feed. This type of farming and husbandry is an FDA-regulated industry that originated in the 1940s. By the 1960s it was known as "the green revolution." "Organic" foods exclude all genetically modified organisms, or GMOs. Genetic modification is a process designed to make plants resist pests, tolerate herbicides, and survive weather changes, all in the interest of increasing crop yield.

What's the Difference?

A 2013 Stanford University study—actually an analysis of 237 previous studies—found no substantial differences between organic and conventional foods in terms of nutrient levels as well as bacterial and fungal contamination. However, the team did find an important difference in the levels of pesticides—and that alone is enough to convince many people to buy organic.

The researchers found that only 7% of organic foods had detectable pesticide residue, presumably because of contamination from nearby fields. Yet a whopping 38% of conventionally grown food had pesticide residue. The study also showed that the two groups of food had about the same levels of E. coli bacteria, which can cause serious illness and even death.

A Quandary at the Supermarket

Organic foods, once found only in health food stores, are now staples at most supermarkets. You stroll through the produce department of your favorite grocery store looking for, say, pears and apples. Do you choose conventionally grown items or organic ones? Both are nutritious. Both provide plenty of vitamins and fiber. You have no way of knowing how much pesticide residue each contains. Do you go with the odds that the organic versions will be cleaner? Do you go by appearance? Organic fruits and vegetables often don't look perfect; they may have unusual shapes and colors and be smaller than their conventional counterparts. Or do you decide based on cost? Conventionally grown produce typically costs less, but are the savings worthwhile? Are you sacrificing safety? Is the organic produce really more nutritious, despite the findings of the Stanford University study?

There are no definitive answers to those questions, but keep in mind that organic foods are even more strictly regulated than conventional foods. The U.S. Department of Agriculture (USDA) has established an organic certification program that requires all organic foods to meet rigorous government standards. These standards control how such foods are grown, handled, and processed.

ORGANIC LABELING

The label on an organic product tells you a lot about that product. Here is what you need to know about organic labeling:

- A product labeled as organic must be USDA-certified unless the producer sells no more than $5,000 a year in organic foods.
- Even the smaller producers must follow the USDA's standards for organic foods.
- The USDA Organic seal is voluntary, but most producers display it.
- Single-ingredient foods such as fruits, vegetables, and eggs can be labeled "100% organic."

- Foods with multiple ingredients such as breakfast cereals and packaged mixes must specify whether or not they are "100% organic" or simply "organic," which is the case if they only have up to 95% organic ingredients.
- Products with at least 70% organic ingredients may say "made with organic ingredients" on the label and are not permitted to use the USDA seal.
- Products with less than 70% organic ingredients are not allowed to use the USDA seal or the word "organic" when referring to the entire product on their labels, but they may list the organic ingredients.

NATURAL VS. ORGANIC

Don't assume that "natural" means the same as "organic." As I just explained, the word "organic" on a label means something very specific. That's not the case with "natural." Keep in mind that food manufacturers use food labels to get your attention. A label such as "100% natural" or "all natural" makes the food seem so wholesome, healthful, and nutritious, doesn't it? However, the word "natural" hasn't been well defined and isn't routinely regulated by any government department.

This is the FDA's stated policy: "From a food science perspective, it is difficult to define a food product that is 'natural' because the food has probably been processed and is no longer the product of the earth. That said, FDA has not developed a definition for use of the term natural or its derivatives. However, the agency has not objected to the use of the term if the food does not contain added color, artificial flavors, or synthetic substances."

The USDA does regulate the use of the word "natural," but only for the labeling of meat, poultry, and eggs. It means that the product contains no artificial ingredients or added colors and is only "minimally processed," although the specifics of processing are not defined. Worse from the standpoint of the consumer, the meat, poultry, or eggs may contain hormones or antibiotics.

The FDA and USDA policies obviously give the food industry tremendous leeway. Unhealthy foods could be labeled "natural." GMO foods could also bear that label. So could foods containing high fructose corn syrup. Or meat containing antibiotics. Such products, needless to say, would derail your Candida Cleanse diet, so read the ingredients on labels and don't fall for the designation of "natural."

To recap, you are not required to use organic foods on the Candida Cleanse, but you may be wise to opt for organic. Weigh all of the considerations outlined in this chapter and make your own decision. The acid test, of course, is whether eating conventional foods fails to make you feel better. If that is the case, try organic—but not "natural"—foods and see if your cleanse becomes more effective.

While we're discussing what types of food to buy for your diet, we also need to compare fresh, frozen, and canned fruits and vegetables. If you've always thought fresh produce is superior, what you learn in the next chapter may surprise you!

13

Fruits and Vegetables: Fresh vs. Frozen and Canned

You can thank Ronald Reagan for the fact that March is officially Frozen Food Month. Back in 1984, the president, issued a proclamation designating March 6 as Frozen Food Day. This odd observance stemmed from his fondness for TV dinners. The day has since expanded to embrace the entire month of March, which also happens to be National Nutrition Month.

Somewhat surprisingly, that juxtaposition turns out to be fitting. Plenty of people assume that fresh produce is healthier than the frozen and canned versions, but that's not always the case. Flash-frozen fruits and vegetables are actually better for you than most fresh produce. The same goes for many canned vegetables if the salt content is low, and for many canned fruits if no sugary syrups are added. (Tip: Rinse canned vegetables to lower the salt content, and buy canned fruits packed in their own juice.)

Why Frozen and Canned Products Are Healthy

Fruits and vegetables that end up in your supermarket were almost always picked before they were ripe, so they never reached their full nutrient potential. Adding to the problem, the antioxidant content gradually diminishes when the produce is shipped and while it sits in a store waiting for you to buy it. Unless you grow your own veggies and fruits or you frequent farmers markets and stop at roadside farm stands, you're better off buying produce that was flash-frozen or canned at peak nutrition. That means the produce needs to be frozen or canned right after being harvested, before its nutrients begin to degrade. A 2007 study at the University of California, Davis found that the loss of nutrients in fresh products during storage may be even more significant than most people realize and that exclusive recommendations of fresh produce ignored the nutrient benefits of canned and frozen foods.

In 2006, the American Dietetic Association, since renamed the Academy of Nutrition and Dietetics, came out with a statement in favor of canned fruits and vegetables as good substitutes for fresh produce. It noted that canned produce might sometimes be healthier because it's picked and canned at peak freshness. Heating during canning does destroy some vitamins, but most of the nutrients remain. The statement went on to say that—as a result of the canning process—canned tomatoes, corn, and carrots provide higher levels of some antioxidants than their fresh counterparts.

Keep in mind also that the nutritional value of fresh produce varies depending on the season. In Mediterranean countries, for example, people generally eat only local produce during the time of year each fruit or vegetable is available. In the United States, however, shoppers take it for granted that produce will be brought in all year round from

AN INTERESTING ASIDE

The commercial frozen food industry was invented in the 1920s by Clarence Birdseye (his real name!), who got the idea while on fur-trapping expeditions to Labrador some years previously. He observed that the local native people froze food to preserve it, and thus an industry was born. By 1998, the FDA confirmed that frozen produce offers the same essential nutrients that fresh-picked produce does.

far-flung areas of the country or indeed the world. Because of this practice, we have an abundance of choices every day of the year but few of us realize that the bulk of what's available is not really "fresh" anymore. Nutrients including thiamine and vitamins A and C are often destroyed by the time we buy the produce. Some veggies and fruits do continue to ripen after they are picked, but they never reach full nutrient value if they weren't ripe when they were harvested.

I'm not suggesting that you should only buy locally grown produce. After all, the lemons in the produce section of your supermarket weren't grown in your state unless you live in one of a few states. And of course, you can't buy canned or frozen lemons. Even so, when it comes to many fruits and vegetables, you may be better off heading for the freezer section of the supermarket as well as the aisles containing canned foods during seasons when your home state isn't producing much variety.

HOME FREEZING AND CANNING

Of course, you could can and freeze your own fruits and vegetables, but those are time-consuming projects. Also, amateurs are not always successful when it comes to preserving food safely. If you learned the art of canning at your mother's or grandmother's knee, go for it. Otherwise, you are probably better off leaving the canning and freezing to the pros.

Getting the Most Out of Frozen and Canned Foods

Here's a guide to getting the maximum nutritional benefit from flash-frozen and canned foods:

- Stay away from vegetables smothered in high-calorie sauces.
- Read labels to find products with low amounts of sodium and sugar.
- Look for the USDA "U.S. Fancy" shield instead of the lower grades "U.S. No. 1" and "U.S. No. 2."
- Avoid dented or bulging cans, which can mean the contents are contaminated.
- Make sure your freezer is always set to 0°F (-18°C).

Remember that raw veggies and fruits are not necessarily superior to cooked. Heat releases nutrients and makes them easier to absorb, so canned vegetables—which by definition have been cooked—can be more nutritious than fresh vegetables. Just be sure not to overheat the veggies after you open the cans. Warm them but don't boil them.

Frozen Foods to Avoid

Keep in mind that when you head to the frozen food aisle in search of fruits and veggies, you may be tempted by the nearby displays of frozen foods that are forbidden on the 21-day Candida Cleanse and subsequent phases of the diet. Promise yourself you'll walk right past the packaged frozen dinners, even the ones labeled "light" or "healthy," because they contain all kinds of preservatives you don't want to ingest and probably a lot of sodium and sugar as well. And it goes without saying that you won't even go near the sugar-laden frozen desserts that would feed the fungus. Right? Right!

Now, let's move on to a discussion of how certain lifestyle changes can boost the effectiveness of the Candida Cleanse.

14
What About My Lifestyle in General?

The Candida Cleanse is going to make you feel a lot better but in order to reach optimum health, you need to pay attention to other aspects of your life in addition to diet. Here are some strategies to help you do just that:

Get Regular Exercise

You really need to exercise, especially if you have a desk job and drive or ride to and from work. But maybe the word "exercise" makes you think of boring or grueling workouts you'd rather avoid. Here's some inspiration to help you overcome any reluctance: A study of hospitalized frail elderly at a geriatric rehabilitation unit of a Veterans Affairs hospital and the transitional care unit of a community nursing home found that resistance training produced amazing results. An astonishing two-thirds of the wheelchair-bound participants with a mean age of 82 were able to get up and walk unaided again after just 10 weeks of training with ankle weights! Here are tips on how to get moving:

Start Slowly   If all you do the first day is buy a pair of good sneakers so you can begin a walking regimen, that's progress. Congratulate yourself and vow to put the shoes on the next day and commit to 15 minutes of walking, whether around the block, in a mall, or at a park.

Go Easy at the Beginning   Don't risk injury, exhaustion, and discouragement by doing too much too soon. Chair exercises are a good choice if you've been sedentary for a long time. First, lift ankle weights just like those hospitalized, frail elderly folks I told you about. You can buy the weights at any sports equipment store or on the Internet. Next, do some arm swings and head rolls. You can also invest in graded resistance bands. Use them for arm and leg exercises illustrated in the booklet that comes with the bands. Finally, if you sit on an inflatable exercise ball instead of a chair, so much the better. You'll be forced to use your abdominal and back muscles to maintain your balance.

Pay for a Class   After you've been doing the easy-does-it exercises at home for about a month, consider signing up for lessons. There's nothing like plunking down some money in advance to make yourself go to the sessions. Pick fun activities such as Zumba (aerobic fitness performed to Latin dance music), square dancing, Piloxing (a combination of Pilates, boxing, and dance), or swimming. That way you'll be even more motivated.

Quit Smoking

According to smokefree.gov, one of the keys to successfully quitting is to create a "quit plan." Here's how:

Pick a Quit Date   Choose a date that's 2 weeks away or less. Mark it on your calendar and also post it near your desk or on your refrigerator so you'll be reminded often.

Tell Your Friends and Family   Let everyone important in your life know that you are preparing to quit. You'll have a better chance of success with support from the people you care about and who care about you.

Get Rid of Reminders of Smoking   Throw away ashtrays, matches, and lighters, and give your home and car a thorough cleaning. You don't want the smell of smoke to linger and bring back the urge to light up. On the appointed day, toss your last pack of cigarettes.

Consider Joining Cessation Groups or Using Aids   Over-the-counter medications can help. Do consult your doctor, however, before taking any OTC medications. Support groups are valuable as well. One option is SmokefreeTXT, a mobile text messaging service. There are also various apps available. To talk to a live human being for help and encouragement, call 1-800-QUIT-NOW (1-800-784-8669).

Get Enough Sleep

Most experts agree that adults need 7 to 9 hours of sleep a night to feel their best and ward off health problems. The National Sleep Foundation says it's best not to rely on sleeping pills. Here are some tips for getting enough zzzs naturally:

- Follow regular sleep and wake schedules even on weekends and holidays.
- Make bedtime relaxing by creating a routine that could include a bubble bath, listening to calming music, or reading—but not on an electronic device. Research has shown that too much screen time can give you insomnia.
- Make sure your bedroom is dark and not too hot.
- Invest in a good mattress and pillow.
- Have your last meal or snack about 3 hours before bedtime.
- Exercise regularly, but not right before you climb into bed.

Lower Your Stress Level

According to the National Institutes of Mental Health (NIMH), everyone feels stressed from time to time, but some people cope with stress more effectively or recover from stressful events more quickly than others. NIMH defines stress as the brain's response to any demand. Many things can trigger this response, including change, whether positive or negative. With chronic stress, chemicals in your body can weaken your immune system and negatively affect your digestive, excretory, and reproductive systems.

Here are some tips that may help you to cope with stress:

- Get help from a mental health care provider if you are truly overwhelmed, have suicidal thoughts, or are self-medicating with drugs or alcohol in order to cope.
- Don't let yourself become isolated. You need a social support network of friends, family, and community or religious organizations.
- Learn to set priorities so that your to-do list doesn't seem impossible.
- Try not to dwell on your problems. Watching a comedy show or a funny movie or simply taking a brisk walk can get your mind off what's worrying you.
- Try meditation, yoga, tai chi, or other gentle exercises.

THE CORTISOL SWITCH

Sara Gottfried, M.D., author of *The Hormone Cure,* says that when you're stressed, you initially feel "the positive vibe of cortisol—the rise of energy, the focus, the charge, the ascent." She explains that cortisol is the main stress hormone made in your adrenal glands and that it's designed to get you out of danger. It raises blood sugar and blood pressure, and modulates immune function.

That all sounds good, but the problem is that eventually your body stops registering the positive aspects of cortisol and switches you to the negative aspects. You get jittery and nervous and your blood sugar drops. Dr. Gottfried reminds us that sustained high cortisol levels are linked to high blood pressure, diabetes, increased belly fat, brain changes such as atrophy of the hippocampus (where memory is synthesized), depression, insomnia, and poor wound healing. Although she's a Harvard-trained physician, Dr. Gottfried admits that she once struggled with high cortisol, pre-diabetes, and extra fat around her midsection. She says that conventional medicine had no answers for her but that she figured out a program that conquered her stress. She recommends the following:

- Eat nutrient-dense foods and avoid refined carbs and sugar.
- Practice mindfulness, the act of focusing your attention and awareness on the present moment. Dr. Gottfried cites a 2011 study at the University of California, San Francisco showing that obese women who stayed with a mindfulness program that teaches sitting meditation, body awareness, and mindful movement for 4 months lost belly fat.

- Practice yoga and Pilates rather than running or jogging.

Now, let's move on to a discussion of how you can prepare yourself psychologically to stay on the diet.

15

Compliance vs. Adherence

You may have noticed that most health care professionals have stopped using the word "compliance" when referring to whether or not people stick with medication regimens or apply sunscreen daily or exercise on a regular basis. The word most often used now is "adherence." The rationale is that telling patients to comply smacks of issuing a command, whereas asking them to adhere implies that they are partners in their care and can use free will to do what's best for their health.

Whether or not that bit of semantic reasoning makes anyone feel more inclined to make lifestyle changes, I believe you can use it to your advantage when following the Candida Cleanse. Instead of feeling punished because you have to comply with the rules, tell yourself that you are *choosing* to adhere to a regimen that will banish your Candida symptoms and restore your vitality and well-being. You are in control—and that means being proud of yourself as well as more forgiving; you're less likely to beat yourself up if you fall off the wagon and have to climb back on.

Why We Overeat and Eat the Wrong Foods

Have you ever wondered why some people—perhaps including you—have a tendency to overeat or eat the wrong foods? Researchers in Germany have discovered the reason for "hedonic hyperphagia," the scientific term for overeating for pleasure rather than hunger.

For the study, lab rats were offered three test foods in addition to their standard rat chow pellets: powdered animal chow, a mixture of fat and carbohydrates, and potato chips. The rats ate all three, but they more actively pursued the potato chips. The scientists used magnetic resonance imaging (MRI) and saw that the rats' brains reacted much more positively to the potato chips than to the other food choices. A long-held belief has been that people and animals want certain foods even when they're not hungry simply because of the high ratio of fats and carbs. But the rats' brains lit up much more in response to the potato chips than to the mixture of fats and carbohydrates they were offered. The reward and addiction centers of the brain were most affected, but there were also differences in other centers of the brain.

Obviously, there is something other than the high ratio of fats and carbs that makes potato chips so desirable to rats—and to people. The study's lead researcher, Tobias Hoch, Ph.D., suggested that the reason some people are able to resist foods like potato chips is that individual taste preferences overrule the reward signal from the food. He also brought up the fact that certain people have more willpower than others. Unfortunately, a lot of us will heed the reward signal and toss willpower out the window. Dr. Hoch believes that if researchers can find the molecular triggers in food that stimulate the reward center, the next step could be developing drugs to block the signal.

Defeat Unhealthy Cravings

Until drugs to block unhealthy cravings are developed, try these strategies to keep yourself from reaching for forbidden sweets or any other food you shouldn't be eating on the Candida Diet.

- **Distract yourself.** If you feel the urge to buy a candy bar when you see the display by the checkout counter at the supermarket, do something quickly to get your mind off the sweet treats. You could whip out your cell phone and check your email or the weather. You could start a pleasant conversation with the person who's ringing up your items. You could mentally start trying to count backwards from 100 by sevens, the so-called "serial sevens" test for mental acuity. Any activity that will divert your attention from the candy will help you get past a moment of weakness.

- **Chew gum.** Choose a brand sweetened with xylitol, which dentists recommend. If you're in public, don't forget what your mother probably taught you about chewing with your mouth closed.

- **Lower your stress level.** If you're an "emotional eater" who has always tended to use food to ease anxiety, switch to other ways to calm down such as soaking in a warm bath scented with aromatherapy oils or doing some deep breathing by inhaling slowly through your nose and exhaling slowly through your mouth.

- **Don't skip meals, especially not breakfast.** Even if you don't feel hungry in the morning, eat a good breakfast consisting of foods on the allowed list for the Candida Diet. If you don't, your blood sugar will drop and you'll probably experiences cravings for sugar or other forbidden carbohydrates. Eat lunch about 4 hours after breakfast, then have a mid-afternoon snack and an early dinner. But resist the temptation to eat before bedtime or indulge in nighttime noshing!

Deal with Disappointment

A study done at INSEAD Business School found that football fans pig out on saturated fats and sugars on Mondays following a big game that their favorite team loses. The lead researcher, Yann Cornil, noted, "Although prior studies had shown that sport outcomes influence reckless driving, heart attacks, and even domestic violence, no one had examined how they influence eating."

The study correlated the outcomes from two years' worth of NFL games with food consumption by fans in more than two dozen cities. The result? On Mondays, fans in cities with a losing team ate about 16% more saturated fat than normal while fans in cities with a winning team ate about 9% less saturated fat than usual. A particularly close game made the trend even more obvious. And when the study included non–football fans in the mix, the trend held.

The researchers surmised that fans—and even non-fans—feel a threat to their identity when their team loses, and they are more apt to use food as a coping mechanism. By comparison, a winning team seems to boost a person's self-control.

WRITE DOWN WHAT MATTERS TO YOU

You may have asked yourself, what about the cities with perennially losing football teams? Do the fans there eat themselves silly every Monday, year after year? The researchers came up with a solution that they tested in their study of NFL fans: After a defeat, fans would down what mattered to them in life. They found that this technique, which they called "self-affirmation," wiped out the effects of losing.

That's a terrific tip whether your reason for wavering in your commitment to Candida-busting eating is a losing football team or any other setback in life.

Avoid Diet Sabotage

Of course, I realize that you are not dieting in a vacuum. You may have young children or a spouse, or perhaps elderly parents or roommates, living with you who sabotage your efforts even without realizing it. Living alone can also work against you: A long-term study in Europe showed that people on their own don't eat as well as people sharing quarters.

Let's look at how to deal with various life scenarios:

- **Parents of young children**—Helping your children learn to eat more vegetables and fewer foods with sugar and white flour is in their best interest. If you start when they're little, you'll have more success. But even if your kids are now tweens and teens, you can gradually accustom them to healthier eating habits. You don't have to keep them from eating the occasional treat, including birthday cake and ice cream, but they really don't need dessert every day. They also don't need candy on a regular basis, and definitely no soft drinks at all. In other words, your Candida Cleanse diet doesn't have to be in conflict with the way the rest of the family eats even if your menus are stricter than theirs.

- **Singles**—You need to discipline yourself to stock up on healthy foods and to cook at home as much as possible. Especially if you're older, you may fall prey to poor eating habits. That was the startling conclusion of the European study I mentioned: Older single adults ate 2.3 fewer servings of vegetables per day than other people did.

- **Caregivers**—You may be so focused on your loved one's welfare that you neglect your own. Don't let that happen! You need to be strong and healthy to be an effective caregiver. Make time to sit down and eat your nutritious Candida-busting meals. If need be, ask a family member or friend to spell you now and then so you can eat better and also lower your stress level. Keep in mind that the fruits, vegetables, and other nutritious fare on the Candida Cleanse diet are good for your loved one as well.

Here are some tips for coping when you're not the one doing the cooking:

- **Eating at restaurants**—Consider requesting a gluten-free menu even if you're not allergic. Also, ask to have your food baked or steamed and to have the chef leave off any sauces. Needless to say, you won't order dessert.

- **Going to parties**—Master the art of "sober socializing." Ask for a club soda and don't make a big deal out of that. Then at the buffet table, head for the nuts, veggies, and allowed fruits and meats. Skip the dips and trays of sweets, and you'll be fine.

- **Eating at corporate functions and conferences**—If there's a vegan or vegetarian option, order it ahead of time even if you're not a vegetarian. That way you won't end up with a plate of food you shouldn't be eating. If there's no vegetarian option, fill up on salad and veggies and don't eat anything with mysterious sauces and ingredients. And whatever you do, wave the server away when he or she comes by with breads and desserts.

- **Being a houseguest**—This can be tricky but you may need to share your dietary needs with your host. You're not asking for weird ingredients, after all. You just need to be sure there will be food on hand that you are allowed to consume.

So, now you're armed with all the strategies you need to adhere to the Candida Cleanse. Even so, picking just the right time to start can mean the difference between success and frustration. Read on to learn how to decide the best time to begin.

16

When Should I Start My Cleanse?

The sooner you begin eating to beat back the fungus, the sooner you'll feel great again, even accounting for a probable little setback during Candida die-off, usually after the 21-day initial phase.

Pick a Starting Date

You may find that sticking to the diet is easier if you start on a date that has positive significance for you—maybe the day you met the love of your life, got your dream job, or closed on your first house. Attaching the start of your cleanse to a time that changed your life for the better can evoke powerful associations that keep you motivated.

TIMES TO AVOID

While a date with positive significance is great, avoid picking an occasion that typically involves celebrating with foods and beverages you shouldn't be consuming now, such as birthday cake or champagne. Also, be sure not to choose an arbitrary date that's several months away. You don't want to wait that long without a good reason.

Here's one good reason to wait: If you're reading this right before the holidays that come one after another beginning in fall, it's best to put off your starting date until the new year. By the time next fall rolls around, you'll be an old hand at eating to feel great, but right now you're probably not up to the challenge of dieting during the feasting season.

Something else to consider: Don't start the Candida Cleanse during a time of the year when you're under more stress than usual. Examples are tax season, the anniversary of the loss of a loved one, and a time when your workload increases, such as when a key colleague goes on vacation. Try not to overeat or load up on junk food and sweets while you're waiting for calmer times. That will only exacerbate your problems and feed your Candida. Simply be as prudent as possible and then start the Candida Cleanse diet in earnest when you're a little more relaxed and more capable of self-control.

Once you're ready, think about the day of the week. You may want to avoid starting on a Saturday or Sunday. For most people, those are days of relaxation and beginning a diet then can feel like punishment. Wait until Monday, the start of the work week for most of us.

MAKE IT A SPECIAL DAY

Once you've decided on the exact date, designate it as "Conquer Candida Day." Then mark your calendar to inaugurate this brand new special occasion, and you're off and running! You can also celebrate the anniversary year by year as you continue to eat for optimal health.

Once you're ready to start the Candida Cleanse, the next step is to stock up on all the foods and beverages you'll need to make the diet a rousing success. See Part II to help you make a shopping list. First though, I want to teach you how to keep a Candida Diet Journal.

Your Candida Diet Journal

Many studies have shown that when you write down what you eat on a daily basis, you're more likely to stick with your program. An added advantage of journaling while you're on the Candida Diet is that you can note your symptoms, especially during Phases 2 and 3 when you will be testing how you react to reintroducing certain foods and beverages that were off the menu during the 21-day Candida Cleanse. You'll be able to tell if a certain food gave you a headache or made you feel groggy, or if you felt perfectly fine after eating it. And you can adjust your diet based on your journal jottings. Tracking your experience with Candida die-off, a process you'll learn more about in Chapter 22, is a good idea as well.

You may want to create your journal on a computer, but many studies have shown that journaling by hand actually increases the benefits because the process of writing with a pen engages parts of your brain that involve learning and memory. Based on those studies, you might decide to go low tech and buy an old-fashioned bound journal.

As you'll see when you look at the example on page 139, your Candida Diet Journal is not the kind of diet journal you might keep if you were intent on weight loss and concerned about calorie counts. Instead, this journal is a way to stay aware of your eating habits and your Candida symptoms, if any, so that you can adjust your regimen for the best results.

You'll find an excerpt from the Phase 1 section of one woman's Candida Diet Journal on page 139. The excerpt from the Phase 2 section of her journal is on page 163, and her Phase 3 excerpt is on page 177. These excerpts will give you an idea of what you could record in your own journal.

PART TWO

THE CANDIDA DIET

Learn about the three phases to optimal health

Phase 1:
The Cleanse

21 Days to Beat Back the Fungus

17

What's on the Menu in the First 21 Days?

Succulent fresh vegetables, steamed to perfection and seasoned with spices...the tantalizing aroma that fills your kitchen when you stir cloves of garlic and chopped onion in extra virgin olive oil over a low flame...salmon fillets, broiled and laced with lemon juice...creamy yogurt topped with bright red cranberries...a broccoli omelet washed down with piping hot green tea...chicken stuffed with olives and almonds roasting in the oven...veal chops broiled with tarragon and thyme as the entrée at your favorite restaurant...a satisfying snack of mixed nuts including almonds, macadamias, and filberts. These are just some of the surprising pleasures you can enjoy during your 21-day Candida Cleanse.

Some sources about eating to defeat Candida overgrowth go into such exhaustive detail that you might easily throw up your hands in exasperation trying to decide what to eat. Do you really need to know, for example, that antelope is permitted in Phase I? Nope! Not to worry, though. The list that follows is thorough but not mind-blowing. You shouldn't have any trouble recognizing the items and stocking up on them at your local supermarket or farmers market.

Protein Palate Pleasers

Just in case you're worried that the Candida Cleanse is a boring "rabbit food" diet, let's start with the enticing roster of hearty (and heart-healthy) choices.

FISH

You've probably received three seemingly conflicting pieces of information or advice about eating seafood and freshwater fish:

- Eat fish at least twice a week.
- A whopping 84% of the world's seafood is contaminated with mercury.
- Overfishing threatens the sustainability of many species.

Beyond the eyeball-grabbing headlines is a simple and reassuring truth: Not only are fish and seafood packed with nutrients, but the choices lowest in mercury are also the most sustainable. So go ahead and eat your "brain food" with no qualms.

Here are the best options (the safest and most sustainable), the next best options, and choices to avoid because they are high in mercury and unsustainable:

Best for You
- Salmon
- Atlantic mackerel from Canada and the United States
- Pacific sardines, caught wild

Next Best Choices
- Albacore tuna from the United States and British Columbia
- Sablefish/black cod from Alaska and British Columbia
- Canned sardines
- Swordfish not from the Mediterranean

To Be Avoided
- Bluefin tuna from the eastern Atlantic
- Gag grouper from the Gulf of Mexico, United States
- Swordfish from the Mediterranean
- Spanish mackerel from the south Atlantic, United States
- Yellowtail flounder from Cape Cod

MEAT

Sharpen those steak knives! Every now and then, you get to enjoy a juicy T-bone or sirloin as long as you don't resort to gas grilling or charcoal broiling, both of which usually involve high heat. These cooking methods can introduce carcinogens. Instead, sauté in olive oil or broil in the oven. But maybe you'd prefer a serving from a standing rib roast or a burger-without-a-bun. No problem! Whatever your preference, a little beef is definitely allowed on the 21-day Candida Cleanse. Pork is off the list for Phase 1 but these other sources of meat as fine:

- Chicken
- Cornish game hen
- Duck
- Goose
- Lamb
- Veal
- Venison
- Buffalo

EGGS

Do you remember the advertising jingle "The incredible edible egg"? The American Egg Board launched its campaign in 1977 in response to the bad rap eggs had gotten because of a study linking them to high cholesterol and heart disease. The song was updated more recently to celebrate the positive scientific take on eggs. The current wisdom is that although eggs do contain fat and cholesterol, the yolk is actually a terrific source of energy and also promotes the absorption of the vitamins A, D, E, and K.

For about 70 calories per egg, you're getting a weight-conscious, good-for-you bargain. So, yes, in moderation you can scramble, poach, and boil eggs even during the 21-day cleanse portion of the diet. Chicken eggs are the obvious choice, but you may want to be a bit daring and try goose, pheasant, and turkey eggs as well, if you can find them.

Veggies for Vim and Vigor

I know I promised you that this isn't a "rabbit food" diet, but vegetables in all their glorious variety are a mainstay of eating to beat back the Candida fungus. Packed with nutrients and fiber, these good carbohydrates are your allies in the quest for well-being. You can literally eat all you want from the following list of greens:

GREENS FOR YOUR SALADS

- Arugula*
- Beet greens
- Bibb lettuce
- Cabbage*
- Chard
- Chicory
- Collard greens*
- Dandelion greens
- Endive
- Escarole
- Kale*
- Mustard greens
- Red leaf lettuce
- Romaine lettuce
- Spinach
- Sprouts
- Watercress*

Members of the cabbage family. See the section on Cruciferous Vegetables section on page 120.

CRUCIFEROUS VEGETABLES

These cabbage-family members are "super veggies" that possess amazing antimicrobial properties and have even been linked to cancer prevention. Some of them are in the greens list, marked with an asterisk. Here are more, including some root vegetables:

- Broccoli
- Brussels sprouts
- Cauliflower
- Parsnips
- Radishes
- Turnips

OTHER VEGGIES TO ENJOY

- Artichokes
- Carrots
- Celery
- Cucumbers
- Spaghetti squash (sparingly, since winter squashes have some sugar)
- Pattypan squash
- Zucchini

NIGHTSHADE VEGETABLES (UNLESS YOU'RE ALLERGIC TO THEM)

- Bell peppers
- Eggplant
- Tomatoes

Legumes

Some anti-Candida diets recommend not eating beans, which technically are legumes, until Phase 2, but there is no evidence that legumes feed the fungus. Legumes also include peas and lentils. As a group, they are a terrific and affordable source of plant carbohydrates, protein, and fiber, so they are on the allowed list for your 21-day Candida Cleanse. There's no end to the goodness of legumes: They are cholesterol-free and contain beneficial fats as well as high amounts of folate, iron, potassium, and magnesium. Enjoy legumes as a hearty, healthy stand-in for meat.

Here's a list of legumes you can have:

- Adzuki beans
- Anasazi beans
- Black beans
- Black-eyed peas
- Chickpeas
  (garbanzo beans)
- Edamame
- Fava beans
- Green beans
- Lentils
- Lima beans
- Red kidney
  beans
- Snow peas
- Soybeans

Of course, each person reacts differently. If you find that legumes are slowing down your progress in beating back the fungus, eliminate them until the end of the initial 21-day period and try reintroducing them in Phase 2 of the cleanse.

Mushrooms

There is a tenacious myth that mushrooms should not be part of an anti-Candida diet because they are fungi. This is simply not true, because Candida overgrowth is not the result of an allergy to fungi. However, certain sufferers report adverse reactions to mushrooms. Again, try them and decide whether or not to include them.

Onions and Garlic

There's a debate about whether these healthy items are vegetables or herbs or even spices, but everyone agrees that they're nutritional powerhouses and valiant fungus fighters.

Garlic contains a sulfur compound called allicin, which has antibacterial and antifungal properties. This very healthy little bulb is also a source of selenium, a mineral that plays an important role in regulating metabolism. In addition, garlic is a source of manganese, vitamin B6, vitamin B12, vitamin C, calcium, tryptophan, phosphorus, and copper.

Onions are cousins of garlic and provide many of same health benefits. They are probiotics and they provide vitamin C, vitamin B6, folic acid, plus some fiber. All varieties are low in calories and have flavonoids that are anti-inflammatory. Whether you eat onions raw or use them in cooked dishes, you'll be getting plenty of flavor as well as essential nutrients. Just be sure to wear goggles when slicing onions so you're eyes won't sting and tear, and use a breath freshener after eating raw onions. Those minor inconveniences are worth the trouble considering all the good you'll get from having onions on the menu!

Fruits That Won't Feed the Fungus

During the initial 21 days of the cleanse, you can enjoy the following low-sugar fruits, albeit sparingly:

- Avocados
- Coconuts
- Cranberries
- Lemons
- Limes
- Olives
- Rhubarb

Nuts (and Seeds) to You!

Not only are nuts and seeds packed with nutrients, but the Candida fungus doesn't feed on these foods. You can eat the following raw nuts and seeds. Avoid those that are roasted or have salt added.

- Almonds
- Brazil nuts
- Filberts
- Macadamia nuts
- Pine nuts
- Pumpkin seeds
- Sesame seeds
- Sunflower seeds
- Walnuts

You can also enjoy the following nut and seed butters:

- Almond nut butter
- Macadamia nut butter
- Sesame seed butter

Drink to Your Health

Here are the permitted beverages:

- Green tea
- Roasted chicory as a coffee substitute
- Kefir
- Unsweetened cranberry juice
- Lemon juice in sparkling soda water
- Lime juice in sparkling soda water

- Plain sparkling
  soda water
- Water

Yogurt

While other dairy products are not allowed on the 21-day Candida Cleanse, yogurt is not only permissible but recommended. It contains prebiotics and several probiotics, including lactobacillus bacteria, that help in your battle against Candida overgrowth. Also, the lactic acid in yogurt acts as an antifungal. Read labels to be sure the yogurt you buy doesn't have unwanted additives, especially sugar or artificial sweeteners. Buy plain Greek yogurt. Two good brands are Vaalia and Chobani.

Yogurt is your friend in the fight against Candida, but it offers a host of other health benefits. It can help lower LDL (bad) cholesterol and raise HDL (good) cholesterol, reduce the risk of vaginal yeast infections, and help pare off pounds. Yogurt also guards against ulcers by reducing the amount of the *Helicobacter pylori* bacterium found in the intestines. That bacterium contributes to the development of ulcers and interferes with the immune system. Yogurt is a win-win addition to your diet.

Oils

The two best oils for your Candida Cleanse diet are olive oil and coconut oil. Use them for cooking as well as in salad dressings. They will help keep the fungus in check while doing your heart good.

You may have thought that other vegetable oils labeled as heart-healthy or cholesterol-lowering are just as good for you. However, a study by researchers at the University of Toronto and Western University in London, Ontario, has shown that polyunsaturated vegetable oils such as corn oil and safflower oil actually raise the risk of heart disease because they contain omega-6 fatty acids but hardly any omega-3s. The researchers noted that over the years many consumers have replaced saturated animal fats such as butter and lard with polyunsaturated vegetable oils in the belief that the oils are healthier. The problem is the unhealthy high ratio of omega-6s to omega-3s in the polyunsaturated oils.

The Spice of Life

Feel free to use any spices and herbs (but *not* herbal supplements) during your 21-day Candida Cleanse and beyond. If you don't already cook with spices and herbs, you'll be amazed at how they liven up bland dishes and make eating a real pleasure—without sugar or salt! These are some of the spices and herbs I recommend:

- Basil
- Bay leaves
- Black pepper
- Cayenne pepper
- Chili powder
- Cinnamon
- Cloves
- Cumin

- Curry powder
- Dill
- Ginger
- Nutmeg
- Oregano
- Paprika
- Rosemary
- Saffron
- Tarragon
- Thyme
- Turmeric

After reviewing the ample variety of permitted foods for the 21-day Candida Cleanse, you should feel pretty good about moving forward with the diet. What's even more important than knowing what you can eat is learning which foods and beverages to avoid for the 21 days and which to forego pretty much forever. Those lists are up next.

18

What's Temporarily Off the Menu?

During the 21-day Candida Cleanse, you must steer clear of some items that you'll be able to reintroduce later on a trial-and-error basis. What's so wonderful is that when you read the following list, you can think positively about how you'll be able to enjoy these staples and treats in less than a month! One woman put it this way:

> I decided that the temporarily forbidden foods would be the proverbial carrot in front of my nose instead of regarding not being able to eat them for 3 weeks as some kind of a punishment. I wanted to stay totally positive about my 21-day Candida Cleanse and about the phase that would follow. My strategy was to put the list of temporary no-nos on my refrigerator door. I would look at it and think, okay, in just 3 weeks I'll be able to enjoy these items again! How cool is that? I also did a countdown on the calendar on my computer so that I knew every

morning exactly how many more days it would be before I could have a nice, crunchy apple or a juicy pork chop or a side of brown rice.

Honestly, I never felt deprived even for a minute! True, I also knew that there were foods and beverages I would probably never be able to reintroduce, but once I started feeling so much better during the 21-day cleanse, I didn't even want to go back to my old eating habits!

With that testimonial as motivation, let's look at the foods that you'll need to pass up for just 21 days.

Fruits

They're nutritious and satisfying, but most contain a lot of sugar, which is exactly what your marauding Candida needs in order to flourish. The less sugar your Candida has to eat during the 21-day Candida Cleanse, the better. That means, during Phase 1, avoid the following:

- Apples
- Apricots
- Blueberries
- Grapefruit
- Peaches
- Pears
- Pineapple
- Plums
- Raspberries
- Strawberries

Remember, you're not completely cut off from fruit in the first 21 days. You can have the following, although sparingly: avocados, coconuts, cranberries, lemons, limes, olives, and rhubarb.

Vegetables

Most veggies are ideal for the first 21 days as well as for Phases 2 and 3, because they are packed with nutrients, fiber, and good carbohydrates. Best of all, your Candida doesn't feed on them at all. However, the following starchy vegetables are possible fodder for Candida and therefore off limits for now:

- Beets
- Corn
- Parsnips
- Potatoes
- Pumpkin
- Squash (except spaghetti squash, zucchini, and pattypan)
- Sweet potatoes
- Yams

Meat

The only meat not allowed at this stage is pork. All the rest—beef, veal, lamb, buffalo, venison, and poultry—are fine. If you usually enjoy pork chops, or crown roast of pork, just wait a few weeks and you can indulge again.

Grains

All grains, even those that are gluten free, are off limits for the first 21 days. Because grains are such terrific sources of fiber, you'll need to amp up your intake of low-carbohydrate vegetables on the allowed list (page 119) in order to avoid constipation. Here are the grains to avoid at this stage:

- Barley
- Buckwheat
- Cornmeal
- Millet
- Oats
- Quinoa
- Rice
- Rye
- Wheat

Naturally, if you can't have grains, then you can't have grain products. That means no breakfast cereals or pasta. However, as you'll see when we get to the menus for the first 21-days, there are plenty of other good options, such as yogurt with nuts or eggs instead of cereal, and spaghetti squash "pasta" or eggplant "lasagna" in place of pasta made from dough.

Alcohol

You definitely don't want to have any cocktails made with sugar—not now, not ever. The same goes for sweet or dessert wines. If you have a gluten allergy, beer is also off limits permanently because it's made from wheat. However, although you may be able to enjoy wine, beer, and hard liquor again after the initial cleanse, you shouldn't raise a glass at all during the first 21 days of the diet. See Chapter 11 for more information on Candida and alcohol.

Cheese

Cheese lovers, don't despair! The prohibition against cheese during the first 21 days will be lifted soon enough.

You'll be able to introduce a few select types of cheeses in Phase 2, but for now all cheese is forbidden.

Coffee

Candida can't feed on your morning cup of joe, but you need to forgo coffee during the first 21 days. See Chapter 11 for details on caffeine and Candida.

Vinegar

During Phase 2 of the diet, you'll be able to use an olive oil and apple cider vinegar dressing on your salads. For now, stick with dressings made from olive oil with either lemon juice, lime juice, or yogurt. Those options are tasty and easy to make, so you should be fine. Just look forward to reintroducing vinegar—a true health food—in a very short time.

Okay, you now have the entire list of temporarily forbidden items. That's not so terrible, is it? Let's move on to the list of food and beverages that you may need to eliminate permanently from your diet in order to keep Candida from ever regaining a foothold in your system.

19

What's Off the Menu Pretty Much Forever?

Certain foods are absolutely off limits not only in the first 21 days of the Candida Diet, but also in Phases 2 and 3. As you'll see later, in Phase 3 you may be able to tolerate limited amounts of these bad guys on special occasions, but in general you'll need to avoid them altogether. The chief offenders are sugar and white flour, but you'll lose your sweet tooth and your hankering for hot dog buns made with white flour before you know it!

Here's what happened to one overgrowth sufferer:

My mom decided to visit me for my 30th birthday not long after my husband and two-year-old daughter and I moved from Ohio to California. He had landed a tech job in Silicon Valley and I'll admit that I was kind of disoriented and lonely at first. I was really looking forward to having "Ma-maw," as my daughter calls my mother, come to celebrate with us. When I was growing up, we always baked and decorated birthday cakes for each person in the family. We would pick a theme. I wanted to carry on that tradition. One year my cake was a "stage" for ballerina figurines because I loved my ballet lessons. That same year, my brother had a Spiderman cake. It was so much fun and we each felt so special!

I promised myself I wouldn't eat any of my 30th birthday cake because I had given up sugar two weeks earlier in order to fight Candida overgrowth. My plan was to go to the store with my mom and daughter and pick out cake decorations for a "California girl" theme. Then we would bake the cake and I would turn down my slice when the time came.

So much for good intentions! Not only did I give in to the festive feeling of the party and eat my slice, I actually sneaked back to the kitchen after everyone else was asleep and ate almost the whole rest of the cake complete with gobs of frosting. Was I ever sorry! I woke up the next morning with my old full-on Candida symptoms–nausea, a dry mouth, mental fog, post-nasal drip, the whole bit. I had undone all the good I'd accomplished during the previous two weeks of being a good girl on the diet. Needless to say, I went back on the diet right away and stuck with it. I was fine again in a couple of weeks and I haven't fallen off the wagon ever again in the two years since then.

Forbidden Foods

Here are the items to avoid once you start the cleanse and in the future:

SUGAR

A cardinal rule: Sugar, except for that which occurs naturally in the allowed foods on the lists, is forbidden—even types touted as healthier, such as honey and brown sugar. That's because sugar is exactly what Candida gobbles up in order to keep growing. This is the first and most important tenet of the Candida Cleanse diet. What's interesting is that if you have Candida overgrowth, you may experience cravings for sugar. That's your fungus calling. Ignore it! No more donuts or candy or sweet desserts. Indulging just isn't worth it. You want to kill off the fungus, not succumb to its pleading for more and more sugar.

The good news is that when you cut out sugar to kill the fungus, you will also be doing yourself a big favor in terms of your overall health and well-being.

WHITE FLOUR

Grains are good for you after Phase 1, but when those grains are stripped of their nutrient-laden husks in order to make white flour, you are essentially consuming useless food that also feeds your Candida. I remember as a child being fascinated by Johanna Spyri's novel *Heidi*. The 10-year-old orphan and heroine of the tale yearned for the white bread rich people ate instead of the brown bread her grandfather served. Little did she know that her bread was far better for her than the wealthy kids' bread!

Promise yourself you'll eat only whole grains once you get past the first 21 days. That means brown rice, whole grain cereals that are not made with maple syrup, honey, or other sweeteners, and whole grain bread made with no sugar. No more white flour hamburger buns, hot dog buns, English muffins, donuts, cronuts, cake, cupcakes, white pasta, white rice, or anything else made from nutrient-poor white flour, not to mention added sugar since only very small amounts of sugar are allowed. Your body, your brain, and your spirit will thank you, and your Candida will give up the fight.

PROCESSED FOODS

Typically loaded with unhealthy additives and preservatives, processed foods don't do your overall health any good—although they do provide fuel for your Candida overgrowth. The list includes ketchup, mayonnaise, soy sauce, jams, jellies, frozen dinners (even the "diet" or "lite" versions), frozen vegetables with sauces, and any other products with questionable ingredients to prolong shelf life.

FAST FOOD AND JUNK FOOD

Meals at chains such as McDonald's, Burger King, and Taco Bell are notoriously poor choices and they almost certainly contain sugar and white flour, so give up the habit now if you have it. Ditto when it comes to chips of any kind, butter-laden popcorn, deep-fried french fries no matter where you get them or how they're made, and any other foods that aren't wholesome and good for you.

COW'S MILK DAIRY PRODUCTS

Except for yogurt, skip all products made with cow's milk.

DRIED FRUITS

Raisins, "craisins," dried apricots, prunes, and other dried fruits are forbidden because they usually have high concentrations of sugar.

Stock Your Pantry for Success

Now that you know which foods and beverages are allowed and which are not, stock up so you have everything you need to make your battle against Candida a rousing success.

First, get rid of any items that aren't permitted. You may want to donate canned soups, packaged mixes, and other non-perishables to a food bank. But don't feel guilty about tossing out items such as boxes of donuts and bottles of soda that aren't good for anyone's health.

Next, make a shopping list. Be sure to eat a little something before you go to the store. If you don't have anything healthy on hand, pay for some unsalted almonds as soon as you get to the store and eat them right there. The old adage about never going grocery shopping on an empty stomach is backed by research from Cornell University. In a simulated store, hungry participants bought 18.6% more food, including 31% more high-calorie snacks. Next, the researchers observed shoppers at a real grocery store right after lunchtime and a different group right before dinnertime. The people who had just eaten lunch made healthier choices and purchased fewer items than the folks whose stomachs were growling for dinner. So don't let hunger pangs do you in before you even start your diet.

When you get back from the store with your Candida-busting foods and beverages, you'll be all set to start your Candida Cleanse. Next up are 21 days of sample menus.

20
Menus for Phase 1

These 21 days of menus for Phase 1 of the Candida Cleanse use only the allowed foods. Feel free to make substitutions as long as you stick to the permitted lists (see pages 116–126) and don't overdo red meat and eggs. Also, consider brown bagging your lunch, including salads, especially if you have access to a refrigerator at work. That way you won't be tempted to order fast food.

As with any diet, be sure to check with your personal physician and possibly a nutritionist to make sure you'll be getting sufficient nutrients and calories for your height, weight, age, and activity level. Your doctor can also advise you about special precautions if you have medical conditions and take medications.

Now is the time to start using the Candida Diet Journal you learned about in Chapter 16. To give you an idea of what you might want to record, here's an excerpt from one womans Phase 1 Candida Diet Journal:

Menus for Phase 1

DATE	CANDIDA SYMPTOMS?	NOTES
Monday, June 9	Still feel "spacey" and vaguely nauseous. Also have to keep clearing my throat. Guess I can't expect to get well in one day!	Ate only Phase 1 foods
Tuesday, June 10	Thinking a little more clearly. Wow! Progress already! But still kind of sick to my stomach and have mucus in my throat.	Ate only Phase 1 foods
Wednesday, June 11	Feel pretty good but I miss my old way of eating! I want an ice cream cone. It's a beautiful June day! But I'm determined to stick to the diet.	Ate only Phase 1 foods
Thursday, June 12	Lots more energy! Mucus not as bad.	Caved and had an ice cream cone.
Friday, June 13	Shouldn't have had that ice cream! Talk about live and learn. Feel like I'm back to square 1 with symptoms.	Ate only Phase 1 foods
Saturday, June 14	Still spacey, sick, and mucus-y. Sigh.	Ate only Phase 1 foods
Sunday, June 15	OK, a little better today. Gotta keep the faith and fight that fungus!	Ate only Phase 1 foods
Monday, June 16	A lot better today. I never even noticed before that I always had various mild aches and pains here and there. Now they're gone!	Ate only Phase 1 foods

CANDIDA CLEANSE

Tuesday, June 17	I do have sugar cravings but I'm NOT going to give in. Joined a group of mall walkers for exercise and to distract myself from wanting sweets. Great to have moral support, too!	Ate only Phase 1 foods
Wednesday June 18	Ten days into the 21-Day Candida Cleanse and I definitely am beginning to feel like a new person!	Ate only Phase 1 foods
Thursday, June 19	Still not feeling as good as I would like.	Ate only Phase 1 foods
Friday, June 20	Went to lunch at a fast food place with my co-workers but only had salad. I feel so much better now that I'm getting to the point that I don't even want unhealthy food.	Ate only Phase 1 foods
Saturday, June 21	Bragging alert! I didn't even have cake at my daughter's birthday party yesterday. Feeling fine today as a result!	Ate only Phase 1 foods
Sunday, June 22	For some reason I'm a little tired today and the mucus is back. I guess this just takes time. But I'm better than I was two weeks ago. Onward!	Ate only Phase 1 foods

21-Day Candida Cleanse Menus

Week 1 (Days 1–7)

Monday (Day 1)	
Breakfast	• Plain yogurt topped with fresh cranberries • Green tea
Lunch	• Salad of mixed greens of your choice, grilled chicken, and olives with an olive oil, lemon juice, and garlic powder dressing • Sparkling soda water flavored with lemon or lime
Snack	• Raw almonds
Dinner	• Broiled veal chop with tarragon and thyme • Steamed broccoli and cauliflower with turmeric • Salad of kale and grape tomatoes with an olive oil and plain yogurt dressing • Herbal tea of your choice
Tuesday (Day 2)	
Breakfast	• Two poached eggs • Cucumber slices • Green tea
Lunch	• Warm chicken over arugula and red leaf lettuce with a lemon juice and plain yogurt dressing • Sparkling soda water with unsweetened cranberry juice
Snack	• Hummus (mashed chickpeas) with crudités: raw broccoli, cauliflower, carrots
Dinner	• Broiled salmon fillet with lemon juice and dill • Steamed spinach with nutmeg • Salad of romaine lettuce and tomatoes with an olive oil and lime juice dressing • Herbal tea of your choice

CANDIDA CLEANSE

Wednesday (Day 3)	
Breakfast	• Plain yogurt topped with steamed rhubarb • Green tea
Lunch	• Broccoli and cauliflower omelet • Sliced cucumbers and tomatoes with olive oil • Sparkling soda water flavored with lemon or lime
Snack	• Mixed raw nuts: macadamia nuts, filberts, almonds
Dinner	• Guacamole with crudités: broccoli, cauliflower, carrots • Black beans simmered with garlic, cumin, and oregano • Sizzling strips of chicken, onions, and bell peppers • Herbal tea of your choice
Thursday (Day 4)	
Breakfast	• Plain yogurt topped with fresh cranberries • Green tea
Lunch	• Turkey "wraps" (turkey slices wrapped around lightly steamed vegetables of your choice such as broccoli, turnips, cauliflower, and carrots) • Plain sparkling soda water
Snack	• Raw almond butter with carrot sticks
Dinner	• Broiled lamb chops with garlic, rosemary, and thyme • Steamed brussels sprouts with oregano • Herbal tea of your choice
Friday (Day 5)	
Breakfast	• Two soft-boiled eggs with celery and carrot sticks for dipping • Green tea
Lunch	• Broiled turkey burger-without-a bun • Salad of mixed greens of your choice with an olive oil and plain yogurt dressing
Snack	• Raw pumpkin seeds
Dinner	• Cornish game hen stuffed with olives, garlic cloves, and pearl onions • Steamed spinach with oregano • Herbal tea of your choice

Menus for Phase 1

Saturday (Day 6)	
Breakfast	• Plain yogurt topped with sliced almonds • Green tea
Lunch	• Salad of endive, baby carrots, and canned salmon with a lime juice and plain yogurt dressing • Sparkling soda water with unsweetened cranberry juice
Snack	• Raw sunflower seeds
Dinner	• Broiled T-bone steak, dry rubbed with black pepper and oregano • Salad of greens of your choice, sprouts, and grape tomatoes with an olive oil and lemon juice dressing • Herbal tea of your choice
Sunday (Day 7)	
Brunch	• Broccoli frittata with crushed red pepper and black pepper
Snack	• Frozen plain yogurt (make it yourself by freezing plain yogurt in ice pop molds)
Dinner	• Spaghetti squash "pasta" primavera with steamed carrots, zucchini, onion, and yellow, red, and green bell peppers • Herbal tea of your choice

Week 2 (Days 8–14)

Monday (Day 8)	
Breakfast	• Plain yogurt topped with fresh cranberries • Green tea
Lunch	• Salad of mesclun, olives, and canned salmon with an olive oil, lemon juice, and garlic powder dressing • Sparkling soda water flavored with lemon or lime
Snack	• Raw macadamia nuts
Dinner	• Broiled baby lamb chops with cumin • Collard greens simmered in chicken broth with fennel and garlic • Salad of kale and grape tomatoes with an olive oil and plain yogurt dressing • Herbal tea of your choice
Tuesday (Day 9)	
Breakfast	• Plain yogurt with steamed rhubarb • Green tea
Lunch	• Salad of greens of your choice, scallions, grape tomatoes, and canned albacore tuna with an olive oil and lime juice dressing • Plain sparkling soda water
Snack	• Mixed raw nuts: macadamia nuts, filberts, almonds
Dinner	• Guacamole with crudités: raw broccoli, cauliflower, carrots • Black beans simmered with garlic, cumin, and oregano • Sizzling strips of skirt steak, onion, and bell pepper • Herbal tea of your choice
Wednesday (Day 10)	
Breakfast	• Plain yogurt topped with fresh cranberries
Lunch	• Chicken "wraps" (chicken slices wrapped around lightly steamed vegetables of your choice such as broccoli, brussels sprouts, and turnips) • Plain sparkling soda water

Menus for Phase 1

Snack	• Hummus (mashed chickpeas) with crudités: raw broccoli, cauliflower, carrots
Dinner	• Broiled salmon fillet with lemon juice and dill • Steamed spinach with nutmeg • Salad of romaine lettuce and tomatoes with an olive oil and lime juice dressing • Herbal tea of your choice
Thursday (Day 11)	
Breakfast	• Plain yogurt topped with sliced raw almonds • Green tea
Lunch	• Salad of greens of your choice, scallions, grape tomatoes, and canned salmon with an olive oil and lime juice dressing • Plain sparkling soda water
Snack	• Raw sunflower seeds
Dinner	• Broiled ground chicken burger-without-a-bun • Steamed broccoli and cauliflower with turmeric • Salad of kale, grape tomatoes, and carrots with an olive oil and lemon juice dressing • Herbal tea of your choice
Friday (Day 12)	
Breakfast	• Plain yogurt with steamed rhubarb • Green tea
Lunch	• Chef's salad of romaine and iceberg lettuces, hard-boiled egg slices, chicken chunks, tomato slices, and cucumber slices with an olive oil and lemon juice dressing
Snack	• Raw pine nuts
Dinner	• Roast leg of lamb with fennel, paprika, and cinnamon • Steamed cabbage with bay leaf and garlic • Herbal tea of your choice

CANDIDA CLEANSE

Saturday (Day 13)	
Breakfast	• Two soft-boiled eggs with cucumber strips for dipping • Green tea
Lunch	• Salad of kale, grape tomatoes, and canned sardines with a lemon juice and plain yogurt dressing • Sparkling soda water with unsweetened cranberry juice
Snack	• Raw Brazil nuts
Dinner	• Broiled rib-eye steak with lemon, garlic, onions, and black pepper • Salad of mixed greens, sprouts, radishes, and chickpeas with an olive oil and lemon juice dressing • Herbal tea of your choice
Sunday (Day 14)	
Brunch	• Spinach and mushroom omelet with garlic and black pepper
Snack	• Frozen plain yogurt with cranberry juice (make it yourself by freezing the mixture in ice pop molds)
Dinner	• Eggplant "lasagna" using eggplant strips instead of noodles, with onions, garlic, ground sirloin, black pepper, chopped red bell peppers, and sugarless tomato sauce (stew fresh tomatoes with garlic) • Herbal tea of your choice

Week 3 (Days 15–21)

	Monday (Day 15)
Breakfast	• Plain yogurt topped with fresh cranberries • Green tea
Lunch	• Salad of mesclun, olives, canned albacore tuna, and an olive oil, lime juice, and garlic powder dressing • Sparkling soda water flavored with lemon or lime
Snack	• Raw pumpkin seeds
Dinner	• Broiled ground turkey burger-without-a-bun • Steamed spinach with rosemary • Salad of kale, grape tomatoes, and carrots with an olive oil and lemon juice dressing • Herbal tea of your choice
	Tuesday (Day 16)
Breakfast	• Plain yogurt topped with sliced almonds • Green tea
Lunch	• Salad of greens of your choice, scallions, grape tomatoes, and canned salmon with an olive oil and lime juice dressing • Plain sparkling soda water
Snack	• Raw sunflower seeds
Dinner	• Roast chicken stuffed with olives and onions • Rutabaga mashed with plain yogurt, garlic, and paprika • Salad of mustard greens and tomatoes with an olive oil and plain yogurt dressing • Herbal tea of your choice

CANDIDA CLEANSE

Wednesday (Day 17)	
Breakfast	• Plain yogurt topped with fresh cranberries
Lunch	• Turkey "wraps" (turkey slices wrapped around lightly steamed vegetables of your choice such as broccoli, brussels sprouts, and turnips) • Plain sparkling soda water
Snack	• Tahini (sesame seed butter) with crudités: raw broccoli, cauliflower, carrots
Dinner	• Spaghetti squash "pasta" with vegetables of your choice, chicken chunks, garlic, and onions • Herbal tea of your choice
Thursday (Day 18)	
Breakfast	• Plain yogurt topped with fresh cranberries • Green tea
Lunch	• Cobb salad with mixed greens, hard-boiled egg slices, tomatoes, chicken chunks, and olives with an olive oil and lime juice dressing • Plain sparkling soda water
Snack	• Raw almond butter with carrot sticks
Dinner	• Broiled lamb chops with garlic, rosemary, and thyme • Steamed brussels sprouts with oregano • Herbal tea of your choice
Friday (Day 19)	
Breakfast	• Two soft-boiled eggs with celery and carrot sticks for dipping • Green tea
Lunch	• Broiled ground chicken burger-without-a bun • Salad of mixed greens of your choice with an olive oil and plain yogurt dressing
Snack	• Raw pine nuts
Dinner	• Cornish game hen stuffed with garlic cloves and zucchini • Turnips mashed with yogurt, garlic, and black pepper • Herbal tea of your choice

Saturday (Day 20)	
Breakfast	• Plain yogurt topped with chopped raw macadamia nuts • Green tea
Lunch	• Salad of fresh spinach, tomatoes, baby carrots, and canned sardines with a lime juice and plain yogurt dressing • Sparkling soda water with unsweetened cranberry juice
Snack	• Raw hazelnuts
Dinner	• Broiled hanger steak with thyme and black pepper • Salad of greens of your choice, sprouts, and avocado slices with an olive oil and lemon juice dressing • Herbal tea of your choice
Sunday (Day 21)	
Brunch	• Spinach frittata with garlic, onions, and black pepper
Snack	• Frozen plain yogurt (make it yourself by freezing the yogurt in ice pop molds)
Dinner	• Spaghetti squash "pasta" marinara with sugarless tomato sauce made by stewing fresh tomatoes with garlic • Salad of dandelion greens, grape tomatoes, cucumbers, and carrots with an olive oil and lemon juice dressing • Herbal tea of your choice

Once you have eaten your way through those delicious menus, you have completed the 21-day Candida Cleanse. Congratulations! No doubt you are already feeling like a different person with your overgrowth symptoms subsiding. Now, let's move on to Phase 2, during which you can gradually reintroduce some favorite foods and still keep killing the fungus.

Phase 2:
The Transition

Four Weeks to Add Back
Some Culinary Pleasures

21

What Foods Can I Reintroduce Now?

In Chapter 18, you learned about the foods and beverages temporarily off the menu during your 21-day Candida Cleanse. But don't assume that on Monday morning, on day 22 of your diet, you can suddenly start eating and drinking all of those items. The key to transitioning successfully to a more varied regimen is to introduce new options one at a time in small portions. This is not unlike the way parents introduce solid foods to babies.

You need to be alert to possible problems and stop any item if your Candida symptoms begin to return. Be sure to note your reactions in your Candida Diet Journal. Depending on the length and severity of your original overgrowth, you may or may not be able to include certain foods and beverages right away—or ever. There is no blanket prescription for what you can successfully incorporate into your Phase 2 meals. Only you can tell whether you're still beating back the fungus. Read the questionnaire in

Chapter 2 again to make sure you're not undoing all the good you did on your 21-day cleanse.

Here are some items you can try to reintroduce gradually:

Fruits

These are the trickiest foods to put back on your menu because they contain sugar. True, it's natural rather than refined sugar, but your Candida likes it anyway. However, most people find that if they add these nutritional wonders slowly, they can still keep their Candida overgrowth in check. You might even want to try other fruits such as papayas and mangoes as long as you're careful to note your experiments and your reactions in your Candida Diet Journal.

Apples: Does an apple a day really keep the doctor away? Yes, according to a Cornell University study indicating that the phytochemicals in apple skins offer cancer-fighting and antioxidant benefits. The researchers concluded that eating the actual fruit is far superior to taking supplements sold as antioxidants. Many other studies have found that apples, in particular the skin, help prevent a host of diseases, including liver cancer and heart problems. Given all of that, putting apples back on the menu is probably prudent.

Berries: In recent years, berries have received high marks as "superfoods"—nutrient-rich foods that are extremely beneficial as part of an overall healthy diet.

Blueberries have been crowned as the most "super" of all. Strawberries and raspberries are recommended as well, and now there's a new kid on the block: buffalo berry. It contains large amounts of the antioxidant lycopene and a related acidic compound, methyl-lycopenoate. Growing on trees found on many Indian reservations, the buffalo berry is bright red with a pleasantly tart flavor and has long been used as a source of nutrients by Native Americans. The fruit could soon become a commercial crop, so look for it in your supermarket.

Grapefruit: You can now try either the white or the pink versions of this classic breakfast treat, but don't sprinkle on any sugar. Use stevia if you must, but many people enjoy the tang with no sweetening at all. Warning: Grapefruit interacts adversely with some medications, so ask your doctor and your pharmacist if you need to avoid it while taking certain prescription drugs.

Peaches, pears, plums, and pineapples: Add the four P's of the fruit family to your Phase 2 diet one by one and see if you can tolerate them. If so, lucky you! These juicy and nutritious fresh fruits are great for satisfying your sweet tooth as long as your Candida doesn't thrive on them as well.

Vegetables

You can now try introducing the starchy veggies that were off limits during your 21-day Candida Cleanse. That means you can have the all-American cookout favorite, corn on the cob—but don't drench the corn in butter. Try mixing a little olive oil with salt and pepper and rubbing it onto the corn. Another welcome addition to your meal plans is potatoes, including sweet potatoes and yams for some people. Try them out and note your reactions in your Candida Diet Journal. Tips: Mash potatoes with plain yogurt instead of milk, and top baked potatoes with plain yogurt rather than butter and sour cream. Remember, though, you still can't "have fries with that"! Deep-fried foods are not only forbidden on the Candida Diet but also should be avoided as part of any diet regimen. Other veggies that can make a return engagement now include beets, parsnips, pumpkin (but not baked in a white flour pie crust), all other winter squash varieties, squash, sweet potatoes, and yams (but not cooked with brown sugar).

Meat

Unless you have a religious reason for not eating pork, you can now add this meat to your menu plan. Ham is not okay, however, because it's processed and has added salt. Also, skip bacon, which is high in fat and simply not a good choice.

Grains

White flour and refined grains are still verboten, but you can start enjoying whole grain breakfast cereals, making sandwiches with whole grain breads, and serving sides of such nutrition superstars as quinoa, barley, rye, and brown rice. You'll welcome the extra fiber and flavor. Be careful, though, to read the labels of all commercial products such as packaged cereals and breads and rolls. If the sugar and preservative contents are high, don't put the items in your shopping cart.

Alcohol

The Candida Cleanse diet aside, the current recommendation for alcohol consumption is a maximum of one drink a day for women and two for men. A standard drink is about 6 ounces of wine, 12 ounces of beer, or 1½ ounces of hard liquor such as Scotch. You may be able to indulge in these drinks in moderation. However, you absolutely won't want any sweetened dessert wines and cordials, and you also need to stay away from most cocktails. That includes the increasingly popular margarita, because of both the Cointreau or triple sec and the traditional salt on the rim. Again, only you can decide whether reintroducing alcohol is worth it.

Cheese

Until now, cheese has not been on the menu because you've been avoiding all dairy products except yogurt during the 21-day cleanse and all cow's milk dairy products except yogurt subsequently. You should continue to eschew aged cheeses such as blue cheese, Gorgonzola, aged cheddar, and Roquefort, but you can probably do fine by adding goat cheese, mozzarella (from buffalo milk), and feta (from sheep or goat milk). That opens up the prospect of more interesting omelets and salads and also boosts your protein intake.

Coffee

Java fans, go ahead and try adding coffee back into your daily regimen. If you feel okay, that's wonderful. If not, eliminate the coffee again. This is a very individual matter. See Chapter 11 for more on caffeine.

Vinegar

The best vinegar to add now is apple cider vinegar, which has long had a reputation as a folk remedy for a variety of ailments. It became popular in the United States in the 1950s as a result of the best-selling book *Folk Medicine: A Vermont Doctor's Guide to Good Health* by D. C. Jarvis, M.D. Whether or not the claims of health benefits provided by apple cider vinegar are valid, you'll welcome the chance to mix the vinegar with olive oil for a salad dressing.

All other banished foods are still not permitted. What you do need in Phase 2, however, are antifungal medications and supplements to deal with Candida die-off, a phenomenon explained in the next chapter.

22

What Is Candida Die-Off?

If you followed the 21-day Candida Cleanse to the letter, you are probably experiencing a phenomenon known as Candida die-off. You're killing the fungus, but in the process you may find that the toxins released by the fungus make you feel temporarily worse instead of better. Hang in there! This is the time to introduce one or more of the antifungal medications and supplements described in Chapter 3.

Any medication must be prescribed by your doctor, so make an appointment right away. If your primary care doctor is not a believer in Candida overgrowth, look for another practitioner on your health insurance plan. As for over-the-counter supplements, be careful. They may or may not work, and they may cause unwanted interactions with your prescription meds. Ask your doctor and pharmacist for help.

Why Does It Happen?

Die-off symptoms occur because of your body's reaction to the toxins released by the Candida fungus cells as they die. This resembles the reaction that may occur after you take antibiotics. When the fungus cells are rapidly killed by the cleanse, an estimated 79 toxic by-products begin circulating. Your reaction is highly individual, but classic die-off symptoms include nausea, headaches, fatigue, dizziness, bloating, and brain fog.

If your symptoms are extreme, that means your liver—the main pathway for eliminating toxins—is probably working too hard and you should ease up on your diet restrictions for a few days. Also, if you are having severe die-off symptoms, reduce your intake of probiotics and antifungals for a while.

Hope for Turning off the Fungus

Here's some heartening news: Researchers at Johns Hopkins Medicine and Harvard Medical School have discovered a possible way to turn the Candida fungus from foe to friend. The main stumbling block thus far has been finding a way to control the fungal infection without harming the host—that is, the human being infected with Candida. Fungi are closely related to humans, so most drugs that will kill Candida will also hurt us.

The researchers identified the vacuole—a small cavity or space in the fungal cell—as a point of vulnerability. They discovered that the vacuole needed to become acidic for the fungus to spread, and by stopping the acidification process they could stop Candida's destructive course, with potentially little risk to infected patients.

Previous studies showed that a drug already in use to treat arrhythmia, or irregular heartbeat, had the unexpected effect of blocking acidification of the fungal vacuole. The next step, say the researchers, is to screen drugs already approved by the FDA to increase the repertoire of antifungal agents to combat fungal infections.

Preventing the Fungal Infection

In related news, scientists at Worcester Polytechnic Institute and University of Massachusetts Medical School have discovered a new compound that prevents the first steps of fungal infection. After screening 30,000 chemical compounds in a series of tests with live *Candida albicans,* the most widespread disease-causing fungus in humans, the researchers found one molecule that prevented the yeast from adhering to human cells. Named "filastatin" by the scientists, this molecule now emerges as a candidate for new antifungal drug development.

A bloodstream infection of Candida usually begins with fungal cells attaching to a surface to form a thin layer called a biofilm. Then the yeast cells morph into a form with long filaments that invade surrounding tissues. The researchers found that filastatin curbed the Candida from sticking to surfaces and significantly reduced the transformation of the yeast into the invasive form. Now, research is focused on figuring out exactly what mechanisms filastatin uses in reining in yeast cells.

Consult Your Pharmacist

Until researchers develop new medications to use in the battle against Candida, consider the antifungals described in Chapter 3 and discuss them with your doctor and pharmacist. For the record, I'm a big believer in consulting your pharmacist. Although your first instinct may be to take any and all health care questions to your doctor, keep in mind that pharmacists are actually more knowledgeable about medications. True, doctors diagnose ailments and prescribe medicines to treat them, but pharmacists know all about the chemistry of medications, possible side effects, and interactions with other drugs and OTC products. You'll find, too, that pharmacists are usually very approachable—and you don't have to wait for an appointment!

Not only that, but your pharmacist is a great resource when it comes to antifungal herbs and supplements. If you take prescription medications, always consult your pharmacist before buying any non-prescription drugs or supplements.

Onward now to the expanded menus you can enjoy during Phase 2 as you add new foods yet continue to kill the fungus.

23

Menus for Phase 2

Phase 2 has no specific time frame, unlike the 21 days in Phase 1. For most people, 4 weeks is about right, but you may need to stay at this level for 6 weeks or more if your overgrowth is severe or long-standing. Also, if you move on to Phase 3 and then find that your symptoms are slowly returning, you'll need to return to Phase 2 for a week or so. However, the variety of allowed foods in Phase 2 is pretty impressive, so you probably won't have much trouble sticking with this part of the diet for as many weeks as necessary to keep the fungus at bay.

In Phase 2, you can continue to use all the menus from Phase 1, but you are free to add new options. Mix and match as you please. For example, you could choose a simple Phase 1 breakfast of plain yogurt topped with fresh cranberries and then enjoy a permitted sandwich from Phase 2 for lunch plus a Phase 2 dinner with sides such as potatoes or corn. On the other hand, you might want to do a whole day or two of Phase 1 menus and then a day or two of Phase 2 menus. The key is to pay attention to whether or not you are experiencing any symptoms and adjust if necessary. You'll get the hang of creating your personal version of Phase 2 in no time, especially if you are faithful about keeping track of your eating habits and any resulting symptoms in your Candida Diet Journal. To help you decide what to write, here's an excerpt from one woman's Phase 2 Candida Diet Journal:

DATE	CANDIDA SYMPTOMS?	NOTES
Monday, June 30	None	First day on Phase 2. Kind of nervous because Phase 1 has made me feel so much better in just 21 days. But I went ahead and added quinoa to my dinner menu.
Tuesday, July 1	Still feel good!	I had two cups of coffee this morning. I have really missed coffee! Also had barley with dinner.
Wednesday, July 2	Out of sorts today. That's the only way I can explain it. Was it the coffee?	Went back to Phase 1 foods for today.
Thursday, July 3	Feeling much better.	Had an apple with lunch and also had quinoa with dinner.
Friday, July 4	Feel fine. Maybe I'll be OK with a little fruit!	Went to a Fourth of July BBQ at my sister's house. Corn on the cob was a real treat and I skipped the butter. My sister didn't have olive oil so I ate the corn plain and it was still good. But I couldn't resist the char-broiled burgers. Let's see how I feel tomorrow!

Saturday, July 5	The burger wasn't worth it. Woke up nauseous. I guess red meat is off limits for me, at least for now.	Went back to Phase 1 for today.
Sunday, July 6	Feel better.	Brunch with friends after church. Had an omelet but no cheese. Still afraid to try alcohol so passed on the mimosa. Maybe next week.
Monday, July 7	Feel great.	Phase 2 foods all day and started some antifungals.
Tuesday, July 8	Oops. I think I have Candida Die-off. All my symptoms are back. Better wait on the antifungals, I guess.	Phase 2 foods but not antifungals.
Wednesday July 9	A little better but I know I have die-off. Just have to ride it out.	Phase 2 foods.
Thursday, July 10	Still not feeling right.	Phase 2 foods.
Friday, July 11	I'm hanging in there.	Phase 2 foods.
Saturday, July 12	Feeling a little peppier. Less mucus. Still have die-off brain.	Phase 2 all day.
Sunday, July 13	Quite a bit better! Maybe I've turned a corner!	Brunch but I decided to skip the mimosa again. Don't want to mess up my progress!

A few words about alcohol during Phase 2: Some people are able to tolerate an occasional glass of wine, cocktail made without added sugar, or beer, but not everyone reacts this way. If you want to raise a glass with friends during Phase 2, give it a try and see how you feel the next day. Only you can decide whether imbibing is worth it. If the alcohol seems to agree with you, you can continue to enjoy it now and then. If not, you won't want to impede your progress in beating back the fungus. Wait until you're really ready to move to Phase 3 before trying alcohol again. Even then, you may be like a lot of people who find that drinking just doesn't work for you as part of your continuing battle against Candida. If you pay for any buzz you get from the booze with a return of Candida symptoms, you'll surely opt for the wonderful feeling of well-being from conquering the overgrowth as opposed to the temporary pleasure you might feel after downing a drink.

Now that you're ready to mix and match menus, I have grouped the Phase 2 menus by meal: 10 breakfast menus, 10 lunch menus, 10 snack menus, and 10 dinner menus. Each grouping is aimed at providing maximum variety and flavor while being Candida-unfriendly.

Phase 2 Breakfast Menus

1. Buckwheat pancakes topped with fresh blueberries
    Use any pancake recipe, but substitute buckwheat flour for white flour and plain yogurt or kefir for milk. Use olive oil for cooking.

2. Quinoa pancakes topped with fresh strawberries
    Use any pancake recipe, but substitute quinoa for white flour and almond milk, kefir, or coconut milk for cow's milk. Use olive oil for cooking.

3. Rye pancakes topped with apple slices
    Use any pancake recipe, but substitute rye flour for white flour and yogurt for milk. Use olive oil for cooking.

4. Oatmeal mixed with kefir and raspberries

5. Grapefruit and rice cakes

6. Buckwheat blueberry muffins
    Use any muffin recipe, but substitute buckwheat flour for white flour and plain yogurt for milk or buttermilk.

7. Brown rice cereal (look for Erewhon or Earth's Best) mixed with plain yogurt, kefir, almond milk, or coconut milk and permitted fruits such as berries and peaches

8. Puffed rice cereal (look for Quaker or Arrowhead) mixed with yogurt, kefir, almond milk, or coconut milk and permitted fruits such as berries and pears
    Use puffed rice cereal sparingly because white rice is not as nutritious as brown rice.

9. Goat cheese and broccoli omelet

10. Mozzarella and spinach frittata

Phase 2 Lunch Menus

1. Turkey sandwich on rye bread with lettuce and tomato

2. Salad of mixed greens, goat cheese, olives, and tomatoes with an olive oil and apple cider vinegar dressing

3. Salad of fresh spinach, feta cheese, chickpeas, and grape tomatoes with an olive oil and apple cider vinegar dressing

4. Twice-baked stuffed potato with feta cheese and chopped scallions

5. Fruit salad with blueberries, strawberries, raspberries, and apple slices topped with plain yogurt
   Accompany with rye crisps as long as the label says the product does not contain sugar. Wasa products are a good choice.

6. Chicken and goat cheese sandwich on oat bran bread with mustard greens and tomato slices

7. Homemade chicken soup made with chicken, wild rice, and vegetables of your choice

8. Homemade vegetable soup made with wild rice and vegetables of your choice

9. Asian millet salad with millet, snow peas, garlic, water chestnuts, scallions, and rice vinegar
   Remember, do not add any soy sauce!

10. Corn chowder made with fresh corn, onion, carrot, celery, potato, red bell pepper, and plain yogurt
    Skip the bacon, but you can add chunks of roast pork.

Phase 2 Snack Menus

1. An apple
2. Buffalo mozzarella cheese
3. Almonds
4. Macadamia nuts
5. Walnuts
6. Pumpkin seeds
7. A pear
8. A peach
9. Feta cheese with cucumber slices
10. Hummus (mashed chickpeas) with crudité: raw broccoli, cauliflower, carrots

Phase 2 Dinner Menus

1. Pork chop broiled with apple slices served with boiled red potatoes and corn kernels "creamed" with plain yogurt
2. Baked chicken breast with herbs of your choice, corn on the cob (with olive oil instead of butter), baked barley, and a mixed green salad with an olive oil and apple cider vinegar dressing
3. Corn taco with guacamole, chicken slices, onion, shredded lettuce, and sugar-free salsa made with tomato, onion, red bell pepper, cilantro, lime juice, garlic, and olive oil

4. Broiled T-bone steak with black pepper, mashed potatoes made with plain yogurt and goat cheese, and green string beans with dill and nutmeg

5. Broiled salmon fillet with tarragon, brown rice, and steamed spinach with turmeric

6. Chicken curry made with chicken, curry powder, onion, cloves, garlic, coriander, cumin, and ginger served with wild rice and a mesclun salad dressed with olive oil and apple cider vinegar

7. Pork loin roasted with garlic powder, onion powder, thyme, chives, and new potatoes served with steamed mixed vegetables of your choice

8. Broiled veal chop with thyme and black pepper, quinoa simmered in vegetable broth, and asparagus spears steamed with onion, garlic, parsley, basil, oregano, and thyme

9. Meat loaf made with ground beef, egg, barley flour, and spices of your choice served with a baked potato topped with plain yogurt and a green salad dressed with olive oil and apple cider vinegar

10. Spanish omelet made with eggs, potato, onion, green pepper, and chicken cooked in olive oil and served with collard greens simmered in chicken stock and garlic

After you've worked your way through the Phase 2 menus, feel free to make up some menus of your own. Then when you're ready to give Phase 3 a try, you'll have a Candida-busting repertoire of meals you know you like.

Phase 3: Maintenance

Keeping Candida in Check for a Lifetime

24

Can I Reintroduce Any More Foods?

The answer is "maybe." No part of the Candida Diet is more personal than Phase 3. You, and only you, can find out whether you are able to tolerate any foods beyond what you added in Phase 2. Most people find that the additions they can handle during Phase 3—a phase meant to last for the rest of your life—are very few and are limited to rare occasions only.

As you embark on Phase 3, keep this in mind: The word "diet" can mean a regimen of food you restrict yourself to either to lose weight or for medical reasons, or it can refer to the foods you habitually eat. For the Candida Diet, you must conflate those two meanings into one. Although the Candida Diet is indeed a regimen of food for medical reasons, it is also meant to be the food you habitually eat for the rest of your life. In Phase 3, you will learn what your personal parameters are when it comes to eating somewhat more freely than you did in Phases 1 and 2, without undoing all the good you've accomplished.

Testing One, Two, Three

Here are some items you may want to test as you begin Phase 3 of the Candida Cleanse diet:

AGED CHEESES

Some people can handle cheeses of all kinds, even those made from cow's milk, with absolutely no ill effects. Keep track in your Candida Diet Journal of any symptoms, however, and go back to cheese made from buffalo, sheep, or goat milk if the cow's milk gives you problems. In any case, bear in mind that although cheese has high-quality protein, it is also high in calories. If weight gain is a concern, then don't abuse your newfound privilege as a cheese consumer.

COFFEE

If you had no luck adding coffee during Phase 2, you may fare better at this point. Start with just one cup in the morning and see how that goes. Remember, even studies showing the health benefits of coffee warn that you risk insomnia if you load up on caffeine in the late afternoon and evening. Sleeping well is critical for overall well-being, so why tempt fate? This is an especially important consideration if you are going through menopause and experiencing night sweats that keep you awake. The same goes for men of a certain age who may need to use the bathroom in the middle of the night and then have trouble dozing off again. The key is to decide whether coffee is a plus or a minus in your particular situation and act accordingly.

ALCOHOL

If you didn't try introducing alcohol in Phase 2 or if you did and weren't successful, you may want to give it a go in Phase 3. If you enjoy wine and can handle a moderate amount, feel free to raise a glass. Again, moderation is important. The same studies that show the positive effects of drinking reveal that overuse of alcohol leads to many health problems.

GLUTEN

Unless you have celiac disease or a true gluten allergy, you may want to try wheat products at this stage. Many people who have beaten back the fungus have no problem adding whole grain wheat to their diets. If that is the case for you, you'll have a much broader range of menu possibilities. You'll also find shopping easier because you won't need to look for specialty grains or gluten-free products. The secret as always with Candida is to test your own limits and reactions and adjust your diet accordingly.

NATURAL SWEETENERS

As you now know, your brain is not fooled by fake sugar and any form of natural sugar is food for your Candida. The only alternative sweeteners I've recommended so far are stevia and xylitol. Please use them sparingly since they are in fact sugar and your Candida "knows" that.

If you're someone who really looks forward to sweet treats, you can try insulin powder during Phase 3. This natural extract of tubers and roots is largely soluble fiber but has a small percentage of root sugars. This sweetener gives foods what many people describe as a cotton candy flavor. Some sources of insulin powder are dahlia roots, chicory roots, dandelion roots, and Jerusalem artichokes. Look for the Chicolin brand.

Another possibility is yacón syrup made from the tuberous roots of the yacón plant, which grows in the Andes. The Incas used it as a sweetening agent and so do modern-day people in Peru, Bolivia, and Brazil. The syrup is recommended for diabetics because it doesn't increase blood glucose. It also has antioxidants. Even so, sugar is sugar, so go easy on this option. You can't afford to offer your Candida a meal.

Beware of These Foods

If you were hoping to see ice cream, donuts, hot dogs, and salty snacks among the foods you can try to add in Phase 3, there's good reason those items aren't on the list. Now that you're on a path toward a lifetime of healthy eating, why reintroduce foods that simply aren't good for you? Think twice about consuming the following foods—not just to keep Candida from regaining a foothold, but also because they're downright unhealthy.

High-fat dairy products: Ice cream, whole milk, and cheese made from whole cow's milk have saturated fats as well as some trans fats that can up your chances of cardio-vascular disease and other health problems.

Sweetened Baked Goods: Donuts, cookies, and cake are loaded with sugar, saturated fats, trans fats, and sodium. Best to pass up store-bought versions of these examples of bad carbohydrates. Instead, why not bake your own using healthy ingredients? See Chapter 25 for examples.

White carbohydrates: Bread, pasta, and other products made from white flour have minimal nutrients. The same goes for white rice. You're much better off with whole grain versions.

Processed and high-fat meats: Avoid bacon, ham, pepperoni, salami, hot dogs, and lunch meats. Get your protein from lean sources such as fish, skinless chicken, eggs, and veal. Have fresh red meat only occasionally and be sure to choose lean cuts.

Salt: Current dietary guidelines and the American Heart Association recommend reducing sodium to 1,500 mg per day and not exceeding 2,300 mg per day. But most of us get 1½ teaspoons of salt daily, or about 3,600 mg of sodium. Your body does require some sodium, but too much can raise your blood pressure and therefore up the risk of heart disease and stroke.

Your Phase 3 Journal

Now that you know which foods to test and which to avoid in Phase 3, or the forever phase of the Candida Cleanse diet, I want you to continue the Candida Diet Journal you've been keeping since Phase 1.

Here's an excerpt from one woman's Phase 3 Candida Journal to give you an idea of what to record in yours:

DATE	CANDIDA SYMPTOMS?	NOTES
Monday, September 8	None.	Ate only Phase 2 foods.
Tuesday, September 9	None.	John's 40th birthday. I had a small slice of cake with frosting, a scoop of vanilla ice cream, and a glass of chardonnay.
Wednesday, September 10	Felt a little spacey this morning. Uh oh!	Went back to Phase 1 foods for today.
Thursday, September 11	Feeling better now.	Back to Phase 2 foods again.
Friday, September 12	Feel fine.	Business lunch at a conference. I requested the vegetarian meal just in case the regular meal had hidden sugar, processed foods, etc.
Saturday, September 13	Veggie meal seems to have worked! I'm OK.	Went back to Phase 1 for today just in case.

CANDIDA CLEANSE

Sunday, September 14	Feel fine.	Brunch with John and some friends. Phase 2 foods but I had a "mimosa" made with champagne and lemon juice instead of orange juice.
Monday, September 15	Feel fine! I guess I got away with that mimosa!	Phase 2 foods all day.
Tuesday, September 16	Feel great!	Crazy busy at work. The boss ordered pizza for all of us because we had to stay so late.
Wednesday September 17	Kind of tired today, probably a combination of white flour pizza and the pepperoni plus working so long yesterday.	Went back to Phase 1 for today.
Thursday, September 18	Still not feeling as good as I would like.	Stuck with Phase 1 again today.
Friday, September 19	Back to feeling good again! Whew!	Phase 2 all day.
Saturday, September 20	No symptoms. Feel fine.	Phase 2 all day. A glass of chardonnay with dinner.
Sunday, September 21	Still fine. The wine didn't do me in!	Brunch but I decided to skip the mimosa this week. Don't want to tempt fate!

Okay, so there are certain foods you must eliminate to avoid Candida symptoms, but that doesn't mean you have to follow a Spartan diet (no Mediterranean pun intended) on holidays and special occasions. Let's get to the most enjoyable part of Phase 3: tweaks and tricks that will make holiday and special occasion meals as festive as they ever were, but without allowing Candida overgrowth to gets its hooks in you again.

25
Modifying Special-Occasion Menus

Phase 3 is the time to try some forbidden foods on special occasions to learn whether you are able to tolerate these rare indulgences. If so, that's wonderful. But if not, you'll need to stay on Phase 2 pretty much forever. Still, be thankful that Phase 2 is not a harsh sentence but a fairly easy way to remain in good health and good spirits! The following tips for modifying traditional foods and special-occasion menus will make these meals less risky for you.

Celebrations That Include Cake

Gooey, rich cake made with ingredients on the banned list is the requisite dessert at many festive occasions such as birthdays, showers, and weddings. Some people who have beaten back the fungus are able to have a small slice now and then, especially if they skip the frosting. However, most people who have had Candida overgrowth are unable to tolerate even a little sugar and white flour. If you're a guest, your best bet is to pass up the cake politely. If you're the one throwing the party, you can make a cake using coconut flour, coconut milk, and stevia with almond butter frosting.

Celebrations That Include Pie

If you always have pumpkin and mincemeat pies for Thanksgiving, or cherry and apple pies for other occasions, try making the crust with coconut flour or whole wheat pastry flour instead of white flour. Sweeten the filling with any of the permitted artificial sweeteners discussed in Chapter 11, but test them first to make sure the aftertaste isn't too off-putting, especially if using stevia.

Celebrations with a Roast as the Entrée

You're in luck! Standing rib roast, crown roast of pork, roast turkey, roast goose, a roast duckling, brisket—all of these are absolutely "legal" on your Candida Diet. Just be careful about stuffing, sauces, and garnishes that can add unwanted sugar and carbohydrates. They will feed the fungus. And pass up corned beef. It's loaded with salt, which won't feed the fungus but may raise your blood pressure. Also, skip baked ham for Easter and enjoy crown roast of lamb instead.

Special Sides and Desserts

You'll have to find out for yourself whether or not you can tolerate such holiday fare as potato kugel, ice cream, Yorkshire pudding, and any other goodies made with ingredients that aren't likely to agree with you. Do your best to avoid anything that may have hidden flour or sugar. If you are the host, you can offer these treats to your family and guests and try some yourself. Note the experiment in your Candida Diet Journal and see whether you have any Candida symptoms in the following day or two.

If you do suffer from any symptoms, you'd be wise to pass up the offending items the next time around. There's no need to draw attention to the fact that you're not eating all the dishes on the menu. Most people won't even notice. If someone does ask, just smile and say you feel better when you don't eat that particular food. A detailed explanation about Candida isn't necessary. And if you're the hostess, you can make your own homemade cookies or bars from grains such as oatmeal (using less sugar and omitting unhealthy fats).

Celebrations at Restaurants

Very often an adult birthday, Valentine's Day, New Year's Eve, a wedding anniversary, or simply the weekly date night with your partner or spouse can mean dinner at a restaurant. Start off by asking the waiter not to bring any bread, unless your companion wants some—in which case, you'll have to use your willpower. Another tactic is to ask for any sauce on the side or to specify no sauce at all. At a Mexican restaurant, request corn tacos or tortillas instead of wheat if gluten doesn't agree with you. In fact, many restaurants now have gluten-free menus. Beyond all that, go for broiled or baked entrées such as fish and chicken. Pass up the pastas and skip dessert, but enjoy a glass of wine if you've found that you can tolerate a small amount of alcohol.

Celebrations That Involve Buffets

Usually, a buffet will include platters of veggies and cheeses that you can eat. Skip aged cheeses if you've tried them and noted in your Candida Diet Journal that you don't tolerate them well. Also avoid dips that may contain sugar. If the occasion is a potluck with homemade dishes, avoid casseroles and other concoctions that may have hidden flour and sugar. Most buffets will also have plain sliced meats. Pass up the dessert table and opt for permitted fruits (see page 122). If you simply must have something irresistible from the disallowed list, then take just one small piece. To keep yourself honest, note what you ate in your journal.

Celebrations That Involve Barbecuing

On Memorial Day, the Fourth of July, and Labor Day, ask the designated griller if you can bring your own entrée. You're better off not eating meat cooked on high heat, whether gas-grilled or charcoal-broiled. But go ahead and enjoy the corn on the cob—without butter, of course. Try rubbing seasoned olive oil on the corn for a delicious alternative.

Now that you know how to eat well even during holidays, would you ever want to go back to the way you used to eat before your Candida overgrowth? I'm guessing you are aware by now that the answer is a resounding "no!" but read on to reinforce your willpower and determination to stay free of Candida overgrowth.

26

Why Shouldn't I Go Back to "Normal" Eating?

Simply put, the Western diet, or the prevailing American concept of "normal" eating, is unhealthy. Consuming large quantities of sugar, white flour, and processed foods while leading a sedentary lifestyle has wreaked havoc with our health. Obesity is one result, but even people who maintain a reasonably safe weight can suffer from a plethora of problems, including Candida overgrowth. Studies show that the traditional diets of other regions, notably Asia and the Mediterranean, are much healthier and that when the people in those areas start eating the Western diet, they get sick.

The Asian Diet

The traditional Asian diet includes whole grains, vegetables, and soy products such as tofu. The regimen is low in bad carbohydrates, high in valuable dietary fiber, and packed with essential nutrients such as the protein from tofu and vitamins from the other sources. In those respects, the Asian diet is a lot like the Candida Diet. The exception is that the Candida Diet doesn't allow soy sauce. Unfortunately, this healthy Asian way of eating is becoming less and less prevalent because of the influence of the Western diet worldwide. Harmful elements of the Western diet such as white flour, refined sugar, table salt, and pasteurized dairy products are slipping into the Asian diet.

The effects of the Western diet are all too evident. For example, a 2007 study of 1,500 Asian women found that those who ate a Western-style diet high in meat, white bread, milk, and puddings (a "meat-sweet" diet) were twice as likely to develop breast cancer as a control group eating a "soy-vegetable" diet. The researchers concluded that low consumption of foods typical of a Western diet plus weight control may protect against breast cancer in a traditionally low-risk Asian population that is increasingly adopting the Western diet.

The Mediterranean Diet

Study after study touts the Mediterranean diet as extraordinarily healthy. Common in Mediterranean countries, the diet includes indigenous items such as low-carbohydrate vegetables, olives and olive oil, whole grains, onions, garlic, and goat and sheep cheeses. Sound familiar? Yes, it's a lot

like the Candida Diet, and here are some of the ways it protects the health of the people who eat it:

- By emphasizing vegetables and legumes as
  well as sources of "good fats" like olive oil, the
  Mediterranean diet has been repeatedly linked
  to a reduction in cardiovascular disease and
  cholesterol levels.

- The Mediterranean diet could be the key to living
  not just a healthier life but a longer one, according
  the Nurses' Health Study, one of the longest-
  running studies on women's health and aging.
  Researchers analyzed information given by 10,670
  women in their late 50s and early 60s and found
  that women with healthier diets were more likely
  to live disease-free to 70 and beyond.

- According to a study at the USDA Human
  Nutrition Research Center on Aging at Tufts
  University, the Mediterranean diet may switch off a
  gene that predisposes some people to stroke.

- A study at Ohio State University showed that a
  compound called apigenin, found in many of the
  plant foods in the Mediterranean diet, can keep
  breast cancer cells from being "immortal" so that
  they die the way normal cells do.

- The Mediterranean diet with added extra virgin
  olive oil or mixed nuts appeared to improve the
  brain power of older people better than a low-fat

diet did, according to a study at the University of Navarra in Spain.

- Overweight people who went on a 2-year Mediterranean diet were able to maintain some of their weight loss for an additional 4 years, reported researchers at Ben-Gurion University of the Negev and the Nuclear Research Center in Israel. That diet was more successful than a low-fat or low-carbohydrate eating program.

- The Mediterranean diet may give your brain a boost in addition to trimming your waistline, concluded researchers at the University of Miami and Columbia University. The participants underwent MRI scans to determine small vessel damage, which can lead to heart disease and possibly cognitive disorders such as Alzheimer's disease. The researchers found that the people who followed the Mediterranean diet had fewer brain lesions than those who ate foods higher in fat.

- In a study at the University of Rovira i Virgili in Reus, Spain, researchers found that the Mediterranean diet was more effective than a low-fat diet in fending off type 2 diabetes among 418 adults between the ages of 55 and 80 followed over a 4-year period.

All of that scientific evidence is very good news for anyone following the Candida Diet, since it's so similar to the Mediterranean diet. The new way of eating you've now learned needs to be your regimen of choice going forward, especially if you were a junk food junkie or a sugarholic before you started the Candida Cleanse. And even if you were a fairly healthy eater before, it's a good bet you were consuming fungus-friendly foods without realizing it. Why undo all the good you've accomplished by going back to your previous ways?

But even with the best intentions, many people experience the occasional setback—and it helps to be prepared to spring into action. Read on to find out what to do if you ever experience a flare-up of Candida overgrowth.

27

What If My Symptoms Come Back?

Obviously, if you fall off the wagon for any length of time, you risk having your Candida overgrowth symptoms return. You wouldn't be the first person who went this route, so don't beat yourself up. Learning a whole new way of eating—and sticking with it—is definitely a challenge. Even so, the good health and overall sense of well-being that you experienced when you were able to beat back the fungus should be enough of an incentive to muster your resolve and try again.

I'm going to tell you about some studies of willpower, or self-control, in situations that at first glance may not seem to have much to do with eating to defeat Candida overgrowth—but you'll see that they do. Read carefully and think about how to build your willpower "muscle" with the goal of adhering to the Candida Diet and freeing yourself of Candida symptoms. If you happen to stumble, just start again at the beginning, with the 21-day Candida Cleanse, and give it all you've got this time!

Willpower Plus Unconscious Motivation

You may think that success is simply a matter of self-control, but a study conducted at Technische Universität München, a university in Germany, found that willpower alone is not always enough. You may also need what the researchers call "unconscious motivation," which can influence willpower.

Each participant in the study was given standard psychological tests to assess his or her drive for achievement. Then the researchers assigned the participants a task requiring them to use their willpower. Next, the scientists assigned a second challenging task to determine how much willpower remained. They figured that the stronger a participant's internal motivation, the longer his or her self-control would prevail. In fact, the participants who scored higher in the psychological tests fared better in the tasks.

Similarly, your internal motivation to keep Candida at bay is a key element in successfully defeating your overgrowth problem. Pair that motivation with willpower, and you've increased your chances of long-term success.

Train Yourself to Have Willpower

In another study, researchers at Miriam Hospital's Weight Control and Diabetes Research Center in Rhode Island found that you can train yourself to have more willpower, or self-control, by practicing healthy behaviors.

The research team found that individuals with more willpower lost more weight, were more physically active, consumed fewer calories from fat, and had better attendance at weight loss group meetings. The fact that more willpower led to more weight loss and the other benefits may seem obvious to you—but there's more to the research than that.

The lead researcher, Patricia M. Leahey, Ph.D., likened willpower to building a muscle that gets stronger the more you exercise it. Dr. Leahey led two earlier weight-control studies that included testing participants' overall willpower by having them squeeze a handgrip for as long as possible, through cramping and discomfort. Those who showed greater willpower in the handgrip task also lost more weight, were more physically active, and ate a healthier diet.

Take a lesson from these studies, and think about your motivation to adhere to the Candida Diet. The more motivated you are and the more you exercise your willpower "muscle," the more successful in your journey—and the healthier—you will be.

A Relapse That's Not Your Fault

On the other hand, you may have an overgrowth relapse through no fault of your own, such as when you truly need a long course of potent antibiotics or chemotherapy. Sadly, the same medical miracles that may save your life are almost certainly going to predispose you to rampant Candida overgrowth. Your good bacteria are killed right along with the bacterial infection or the cancer cells that the treatments target, giving Candida the upper hand. Also, if you're a woman who chooses oral birth control, you may end up with Candida overgrowth.

The good news is that in all of these instances, the Candida Cleanse diet can help you emerge as the winner in the battle against the fungus. Just as if you had simply strayed from the regimen and experienced a return of your symptoms, resolve to go back to the very beginning of the cleanse. You already know the drill so the diet should be easier this time around, plus you have already reveled in the wonderful feeling of health you had before your Candida symptoms recurred. I wish you the best of luck!

Now, read on for my final words of encouragement…

Epilogue: Candida Overgrowth, a Blessing in Disguise

You probably picked up this book because you weren't feeling your best. If you had already done some research, you may have begun to suspect that you were suffering from Candida overgrowth. Now, if you faithfully followed the 21-day Candida Cleanse and Phases 2 and 3, you can look back on the days when you were constantly under the weather and give thanks that the fungus was the impetus for turning your life around. Here's one woman's account of this reaction:

> When I first learned about Candida overgrowth, I was feeling really sorry for myself. At the age of 32, I was plagued by so many health problems that I felt like an old lady. That just didn't seem fair! But the more I worked at beating back the fungus, the more I realized that the overgrowth woke me

up to the fact that I needed to make some serious lifestyle changes. The diet was key, of course, but I also stopped making excuses for not exercising, I cut back on the partying, and I quit smoking.

Almost like magic, my stress level went down even though my job as a CPA was as challenging as ever. I was sleeping more soundly too. On my 33rd birthday, I was down two dress sizes and my boyfriend proposed! Looking at that gorgeous rock on my finger, I had no trouble skipping the champagne and birthday cake. Candida had taught me a lesson. If I hadn't had the overgrowth, I might never have known what it's like to feel vibrant and glad to be alive!

Here is one final reminder list that can help you rejoice in your own victory over the fungus:

- Sugar, except for the small amounts that occur naturally in allowed foods, is off the menu for good.
- Sweeteners such as stevia and xylitol are permitted sparingly and only on special occasions.
- Eat lots of low-carbohydrate vegetables for fiber, vitamins, and minerals.
- Eat some fruit, but don't go overboard.
- Eat prebiotics and probiotics.
- Consider cutting out gluten to see whether you feel better without it.
- Drink in moderation or not at all.

- Make a personal decision about whether or not coffee agrees with you.
- Avoid genetically modified foods (GMOs).
- Consider going organic.
- Use flash-frozen and canned fruits and vegetables as well as fresh produce.
- Get regular exercise.
- Don't smoke.
- Get enough sleep but avoid sleeping pills.
- Practice meditation, yoga, and other strategies to lower stress levels.

You may want to copy the list, print it out, and post it on your refrigerator or in your office or cubicle where you'll see it daily—at least until your newfound diet and lifestyle habits are firmly entrenched. Before long, I'm betting that you'll be so well versed in the tenets of the Candida Cleanse diet and so relieved to be feeling well again that nothing could sway you to go back to your old ways. May you continue to celebrate winning the battle against "the fungus among us" as you eat well and take good care of yourself for all the years to come!

Index

Digestive problems, as symptom, 12

Disappointment, and overeating, 105–106

Dried fruits, 136

E

Ear infections, as symptom, 15

Eating out, 107–108, 182–83

Echinacea, 29

Eggs, on diet, 68, 118–19

Electrolytes, and colonics, 33–35

Exercise, 66–67, 94–96

F

Fast food, 136

Fatigue, as symptom, 12

"Female problems," as symptom, 14

Fiber, 43

Filastatin, 159–60

Fish, on diet, 59, 67, 116–17

Fluconazole, 27

Fluids, 44

Food allergies, as symptom, 11–12

Food cravings, 12, 103–104, 134

Foods: avoiding, 117, 127–31, 175–76; on diet, 115–26; forbidden, 132–37; reintroducing, 172–76. *See also specific foods*

Fruits: avoiding, 128; on diet, 58, 122–23; fresh vs. frozen/canned, 88–93; reintroducing, 152–53

Fruits, dried, 136

G

Garlic, on diet, 122

Genital yeast infections, 25–26; tests, 18–19; treatment, 25–26, 30

Gluten, 76–77; reintroducing, 174

Gottfried, Sara, 98–99

Grains: avoiding, 129–30; on diet, 58–59; as forbidden food, 134–35; reintroducing, 154–55

Grapefruits, reintroducing, 153

Green tea, 77

Greens. *See* Vegetables

Gum chewing, 104

"Gut flora," 3–4

Gymnema sylvestre, 30

H

Headaches, as symptom, 13

Hemorrhoids, 38–39

Herbal supplements, 28–31, 157–61

Herbs, on diet, 59, 125–26

Hoch, Tobias, 103

Home colonics, 35–36

Home freezing/canning, 91

Hydration, 44

I

Imidazoles, 26

Indecision, as symptom, 14

Insulin powder, 175

Intestinal peristalsis, 39

Intravenous amphotericin, 27

Invasive candidiasis, 4; tests, 19

J

Jarvis, D. C., 156

Jock itch, 25–26; tests, 18; treatment, 25–26, 30

Journals and journaling, 111–12, 138–40, 163–64, 177–78

Junk food, 136

K

Kefir, 72–73

Kimchi, 73

Klauer, Jane, 77–78

L

Labeling, of organic foods, 84–85

Lamisil, 25, 28

Laxatives, 38

Leahey, Patricia M., 192

Leaky gut syndrome, questionnaire, 19–22

Legumes, on diet, 120–21

Lemon juice, 48

Lemonade Diet, 47–48; risks, 48

Liquid diets, 46; risks, 46–49

Liquor, 80–81; avoiding, 130; reintroducing, 155, 164–65, 174

M

Magnesium, and colonics, 34

Maintenance phase. *See* Phase 3

Malaise, as symptom, 15–17

"Male problems," as symptom, 14

Master Cleanse, 47–48; risks, 48

Meals, skipping, 104

Acknowledgments

My thanks to Ulysses Press editor Keith Riegert for his support and his help in improving this book. I am grateful also for the trust and encouragement of acquisitions editor Katherine Furman, who put her faith in me when she invited me to write *Candida Cleanse*. Deep appreciation as well to Robin Westen, the friend and colleague who recommended me for the project. Finally, a heartfelt thank you to the sharp-eyed and talented editor who did far more than copyedit the manuscript. Susan Lang made excellent changes and she came up with inspired suggestions for making the book the best it can be.

About the Author

A seasoned health writer, **Sondra Forsyth** is the co-editor-in-chief of ThirdAge.com, an AARP blogger, and a winner of the National Magazine Award. Her writing has appeared in *Good Housekeeping*, *Town & Country*, *Redbook*, *Gourmet*, *Cosmopolitan*, *Family Circle*, *Ladies' Home Journal*, and more. She lives in New York City.

CPSIA information can be obtained
at www.ICGtesting.com
Printed in the USA
LVHW02s0449070318
568927LV00001B/1/P